PRANASC

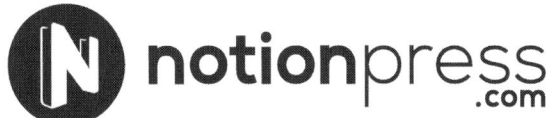

PRANASCIENCE
DECODING YOGA BREATHING

SUNDAR BALASUBRAMANIAN, PhD

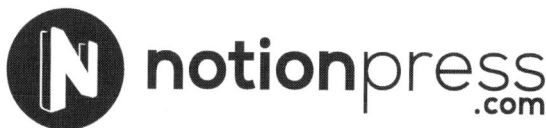

Notion Press

Old No. 38, New No. 6
McNichols Road, Chetpet
Chennai - 600 031

First Published by Notion Press 2017
Copyright © Sundar Balasubramanian 2017
All Rights Reserved.

ISBN 978-1-946515-22-3

This book has been published with all reasonable efforts taken to make the material error-free after the consent of the author. No part of this book shall be used, reproduced in any manner whatsoever without written permission from the author, except in the case of brief quotations embodied in critical articles and reviews.

The Author of this book is solely responsible and liable for its content including but not limited to the views, representations, descriptions, statements, information, opinions and references ["Content"]. The Content of this book shall not constitute or be construed or deemed to reflect the opinion or expression of the Publisher or Editor. Neither the Publisher nor Editor endorse or approve the Content of this book or guarantee the reliability, accuracy or completeness of the Content published herein and do not make any representations or warranties of any kind, express or implied, including but not limited to the implied warranties of merchantability, fitness for a particular purpose. The Publisher and Editor shall not be liable whatsoever for any errors, omissions, whether such errors or omissions result from negligence, accident, or any other cause or claims for loss or damages of any kind, including without limitation, indirect or consequential loss or damage arising out of use, inability to use, or about the reliability, accuracy or sufficiency of the information contained in this book.

DEDICATION

Tamil Sithars
நிறைமொழி மாந்தர்கட்கு

REVIEWS FOR THE RESEARCH WORK OF THE AUTHOR AND HIS TEAM

"Although there is no known cure for Alzheimer's, the following research [by Sundar Balasubramanian] shows how yoga breathing and exercise may help prevent and treat the disease."

Huffington Post

"The researchers [Sundar Balasubramanian and colleagues] found that the breathing exercise group's saliva had significantly lower levels of three cytokines that are associated with inflammation and stress."

New York Times

"From his translation and application of one of the more than 3,000 poems in the ancient script Thirumanthiram, Dr. Balasubramanian, has made an important discovery for public health and offers a simple 1-2-3 exercise for well-being."

TEDxCharleston

"Bobbi Conner talks with Dr. Sundar Balasubramanian about research related to the health benefits of yogic breathing."

South Carolina Public Radio

"Dr. Sundar has committed the bulk of his career to the research of Yogic Breathing and its healing principles." "We are privileged to benefit from Dr. Sundar's groundbreaking research taking place so close to home in South Carolina."

The Colletonian

"A Scientist at the Medical University of South Carolina [Sundar Balasubramanian] has been researching what's in our saliva, and what changes happen during meditation and breathing exercises."

Ashton Szabo, Sivana Podcast

CONTENT EDITORS

Boobalan Pachaiyappan, PhD

Yuvaraj Sambandam, PhD

Payal Shah, B.S.

Devesh Kumar, PhD

CONTENTS

PREFACE .... *xiii*
ACKNOWLEDGEMENTS .... *xvii*

CHAPTER 1
    THE MASTER OF FIVE SENSES 1

CHAPTER 2
    CONTROL THE TWO HORSES 9

CHAPTER 3
    HAPPINESS FROM WITHIN 16

CHAPTER 4
    THE POWER OF PRANAN 22

CHAPTER 5
    THE PRACTICE OF THIRUMOOLAR PRANAYAMAM 26

CHAPTER 6
    WITH BLESSINGS FROM THE GURU 35

CHAPTER 7
    BREATH-HOLDING MAKES YOU A MASTER 42

CHAPTER 8
    KICK THE DEATH AWAY 50

CHAPTER 9
    BLESSINGS FROM A POISON EATER 55

CHAPTER 10
    WHEN A CHANT BECOMES THE BREATH 61

Contents

CHAPTER 11
  NO DEATH 71
CHAPTER 12
  HEALTHY ORGANS AND DIVINITY 79
CHAPTER 13
  THE LENGTH OF THE BREATH 88
CHAPTER 14
  NO DAY NO NIGHT... 93

FURTHER READING 99

PREFACE

It all started sometime in 2006 when I realized that the breathing exercise I was doing, regularly produced more saliva. At that time my family and I were living in Connecticut trying to recover from my father's sudden demise. Balasubramanian Somasundaram, my father, was a middle school principal, but he was widely known to the community as a very soft spoken, kind, and honest man. People turned to him constantly to seek his advice and my father went above and beyond his time to help the needy. I was completely crashed when I received a phone call from my uncle one midnight saying that my father was hospitalized after a heart attack. As I was ready to board the plane in New York to Chennai, I got the news that he just passed away. It happened all of a sudden. I was at the funeral as if everything were to be a dream. I didn't quite feel the heavy loss for about a month during my stay in India immediately following his demise.

Even though I came back to the United States, my heart stayed back home. It was painful to say the least. Who would take care of my mother? My older sister - who herself was a heart patient, would she be able to stay with my mother? Above all, I felt the pain of guilt that arose due to my inability to execute duties as the only son. I questioned myself if I took good care of my father, and why I could not be around him when he needed me the most. The feeling that I never had a final word with him bothered me persistently. I wanted a way-out. This is the time I re-intensified practicing yoga, yoga breathing in particular - that I was practicing on-and-off during the last several years.

Being a Scientist by profession, my curious mind focused on the mechanisms by which yoga breathing works. I launched a one-man's journey towards exploring this several thousand-years old practice. While this noble endeavor helped recover from my father's loss, it instilled a perennial curiosity in me to understanding, practicing and propagating pranayamam (a.k.a, yogic breathing or yoga breathing). The timing could not be any better. We moved to South Carolina in the beginning of September 2006 where I started-off as a Research Instructor in a cardiology lab. In addition to my primary research which is to understand how cells grow and survive stress, I was continuously asking myself why and how breathing practise evolved, and what is its influence on body and mind.

What made me even more curious was the salivary stimulation that followed Thirumoolar's yoga breathing exercise - that too every time I practiced! I decided to explore more in this avenue to unlock the scientific value of pursuing pranayamam. In this journey, Thirumoolar's and several other Sithars' works play a major part. Thirumoolar was one of the earliest Yogis known to the mankind, a Saint from the past. He is quoted as a contemporarian to St. Patanjali. His time is not known exactly. One of Thirumoolar's literary works is Thirumanthiram, a compendium that details pranayamam methods.

My present research work involves understanding the scientific basis of pranayamam, and applying these methods to address unmet medical needs. In addition, I travel to multiple places to teach pranayamam exercises. What I discussed in this book is just a drop of water from the ocean called Thirumanthiram. The book has over 3000 poems, however I have focused on just the fourteen of them because of their direct relevance to pranayamam (Poem # 564-577). By no means I would claim my interpretations are the ultimate ones for this book. I believe this will encourage many to read Thirumanthiram and unearth several practical concepts of life, yoga, devotion, evolution, nature, ethics etc. hidden in this treasure. For simplicity reasons I am not using any italicization throughout the book.

My interpretations to Thirumanthiram are based upon the works of several yoga masters or Saints that I learn from the vast Tamil literature. Tamil is a language spoken by almost 80 million people throughout the world. It is a continuous culture from the ancient past as evidenced by its literature, monuments in India and Sri Lanka (to name just two countries), and by its rich traditional practices. I grew up speaking and writing Tamil and I am fluent to some extent in Tamil literature. This background helped me to understand the wealth of information within the Tamil literature and to become a bridge to transmit the wisdom to others that do not understand Tamil. I hope that this book will lay the foundation for the understanding of pranayamam, and stimulate insightful conversations.

ACKNOWLEDGEMENTS

It is difficult to overstate my sincere respects to Thirumoolar for his revolutionary book Thirumanthiram. I would like to continue to be his student till the end of my time. I gratefully acknowledge the immense inspiration given by my family members, particularly to my mother Saroja Balasubramanian, my wife Janaki, our children Masilan, Nelli and Vetri. They have been very supportive to this ambitious task and has made numerous sacrifices just so I can focus on my work. I could not be luckier to have wonderful in-laws who take pride in my every research endeavor. I am deeply indebted to my teachers (yoga masters, in particular) for the nonstop supply of knowledge, as well as for instilling a perennial curiosity in my mind. I am happy to acknowledge my debt to Dr. Jacobo Mintzer for standing behind me to begin the "first-of-its-kind" clinical trial on yoga breathing. Dr. Graham Warren and South Carolina Clinical and Translational Research have been very supportive for me to continue my research on yoga breathing as well. In addition, several colleagues at the Medical University of South Carolina, Hope Lodge, and the Veterans Affairs Medical Center helped me in multiple ways to disseminate the concept of yoga breathing to the communities. Thanks are due in greater amounts to Pure Action Inc. for their inspiration and financial support. Frequent conversations with my best friends including, Dr. Thangamani Nithyanantham, Dr. Yuvaraj Sambandam and Dr. Santhosh Mani have been very helpful in transforming nebulous concepts to concrete ideas, as well as to present the subject matter in a lucid language for a lay audience. Several thoughts expressed in this book have been pre-vetted by the student attendees of my yoga

Acknowledgements

breathing classes and workshops. I greatly appreciate the discussions, questions and encouragements that resulted from these interactions which provided a strong driving force to write this book. My globally acknowledged TEDx speech in Charleston, and the coverage by several media outlets continue to spread the significance of my pranayamam-based scientific research. I profusely thank the content editors Dr. Boobalan Pachaiyappan, Dr. Yuvaraj Sambandam, Ms. Payal Shah and Dr. Devesh Kumar for their edits, comments and constructive criticisms. The enthusiasm shown by the team at Notion Press (Chennai, India) to print this book is tremendous. I cannot possibly find a press team that is this encouraging.

Last but not least, I would like to recall the immense strides taken by my father to help me evolve as a Scientist - and most importantly - as a person. If I am half as benevolent as he was, I will consider my life a successful one.

CHAPTER 1

THE MASTER OF FIVE SENSES

Original Version (Tamil)

ஐவர்க்கு நாயகன் அவ்வூர்த் தலைமகன்
உய்யக் கொண்டேறும் குதிரை மற்றொண்டுண்டு
மெய்யர்க்குப் பற்றுக் கொடுக்கும் கொடாதுபோய்ப்
பொய்யரைத் துள்ளி விழுத்திடும் தானே.

Transliteration

    Aivarkku nayahan avvoor thalaimahan

    Uyyak konderum kudhirai matrondu

    Meyyarkku patru kodukkum kodaadhupoy

    Poyyarai thulli vizhuthidum thaane.

Translation

    He is the chief of that town

    There is another horse that he climbs towards liberation

    That galloping horse heeds only to the truthful

    The untruthful gets toppled.

This is the first poem under the pranayamam section in the book Thirumanthiram written by St. Thirumoolar. The legend has it that he lived in Tamilnadu, India several centuries ago and was sent by Lord Siva to enlighten the people. It is not the stories about him that inspired me and my research, rather his articulation of the breathing techniques. The above poem succinctly summarizes the ultimate benefit of pranayamam. To be more specific, by controlling the mind it is possible to liberate from the earthly desires. This is a revolutionary thought during its times because even today we are controlled by our mind and it is important to decipher what controls the mind that controls us. Thirumoolar goes beyond and suggests that through the help of its subordinates – five senses – the mind aimlessly wander. For example, the mere smell coming out of a coffee shop draws us from the sidewalk into the cafe and lures us to enjoy a cup of coffee (and, sometimes a nice piece of biscotti). Senses trigger the master (mind) and the latter drives the body. To complete the cycle, our body then feeds the senses and mind. This is called a feedback loop, which can amplify over the time. We can get indulged similarly by all of our other senses. Our brain interprets this information derived from senses, which we experience as life. We think we are satisfied when all the senses are satisfied, but this is only temporary. We are satisfied for the next hour after coming out of the coffee shop. When we continue our walk, we see beautiful paintings in the window of an art gallery, a girl on the street enjoying a walk with her parents, people eating under the umbrellas in front of restaurants, a skateboarder cruising by, giggles of passerby and people with the latest fashion trends. It is important to realize that our senses transmit every piece of information they gather to the mind.

Mind goes after everything, looking at and comparing what you have versus what the body senses outside. For a second we realize 'we' are not the mind. Briefly we get the realization that our mind is an important mediator of us and the world, and a key intermediary between our senses and us. Our mind is not us. Nor, it is the self. But it can make us think that it is the self. The mind is not just a tool like the senses, but a more sophisticated one, that combines all the senses. The mind is a wonderful tool (in fact, a treasure) if it can be conditioned, either be it the determination of Gandhi or Einstein, ordinary people who were made extraordinary by the well-cultivated mind. We have seen several examples in the history of mankind showing the power of mind. Thirukkural is an ancient piece of Tamil literature written more than 2000 years ago and was translated the most next to the Bible. It talks about almost all aspects of life. About mind, Thirukkural says that controlling the five senses (sight, hearing, taste, smell, and touch) within oneself will have a positive impact on life, which in fact constitutes seven segments (life can be of seven stages, for instance the life-cycle of a female is comprised of pethai, pedhumbai, mangai, madandhai, arivai, therivai, and perilampen stages as per the ancient classification in Tamil). Seven could also mean the seven chakras (nerve plexus) that control the function of the whole body. In all these seven stages the control of the mind will bring fame and laurel. Thus, the power of mind can be enriched by controlling the mind, which in turn controls the five senses. However, it is not easy to control the mind. If we cannot control the mind, how are we going to control its downstream cadres, the senses? If we are unable to control the senses, then we are heading towards chaos both internally and externally (social levels). Therefore, controlling the mind is vital to a healthy being.

Just like any other personal preference, every school of thought has a plethora of techniques to practice the control of the mind. For some it is prayer, meditation, or looking into the movements of the mind without being attached to the thoughts or without associating with the thoughts. I asked one of the modern day gurus from India, who often visits the US and goes around the world to talk about yoga. I had the opportunity to share a guesthouse with him once during a yoga retreat. One evening after one of his lectures, I approached him and complimented his talk, as it was full of jokes. Specifically for his light-hearted humor about sudden rise of Yogis, Indian culture, and the stereotypical view of most people about yoga. Interestingly, he did not delve on the concept of controlling the mind. When I asked him how to control the mind, he asked back: "Why do you want to control the mind?" Even though he replied humorously, his words created a revelation in me. I paused for a moment, but asked his opinion about how a common no-Zen man could control his mind. I asked this because I strongly believe that mind is the root cause of all the sufferings that we go through. Then he looked at me after a pause and said, "Put the God in your heart, think about your favorite God, focus on it, and your mind will be controlled." I was not convinced by his answer. I thanked him and left. He did not ask me if I have any other methods. Had he asked I would have told him what I knew. It seems customary for the modern era Swamis to not ask questions or seek answers from others, because that is sometimes perceived as a sign of weakness. They prefer to give only answers! Not just him, but several other masters that I met would rather preach, than listen. In my view, Thirumoolar shows a clear path for mind control, as can be evidenced through this poem.

Mind control, in theory, is very simple and any common person should be able to practice. It begins with a staunch focus on one's breathing. Watch it closely as you begin circulating the air through the nostrils. If your mind wanders, bring the awareness back to the breathing. Breathing is a dynamic activity, yet it allows the mind to stick to it. Let the mind follow the breathing closely. Then the mind won't have anything else to cling onto, and the mind will be far away from worries. Watching the breathing is not a distraction of mind from one to other. Connecting the mind and breathing is not a distraction; it is a retraction within. Once you turn off the switches of the body's lights, the senses get turned off.

The physical body is called Annamaya kottam in the yoga practice. There are five different forms of our being – the physical layer, the breathing layer, the mental layer, the wisdom layer, and the blissful core. Our core nature is bliss. It is covered with the four layers mentioned above. The ultimate goal of one's life is to rise to the blissful state (and remain therein). Next to the physical body is an inner space that is calmer. That place is the breathing layer, or the Pranamaya kottam. Crossing the breathing layer is an important aspect in yoga practice, but often neglected. The yoga practice either stays at the physical level or they directly go to the mental layer to control one's own mind (a.k.a meditation). From within the physical body layer you cannot easily bypass the breathing layer to reach out to the mind directly. That is why Attanga yoga, or the eight-limb practice (consisting of the following eight steps: iyamam, niyamam, asanam, pranayamam, prathyagaram, dharanai, dhyanam, samadhi) emphasizes pranayamam as a critical step between asanam (body) and prathyagaram (a mind practice). As pranayamam is a key practice, the first poem of this section focuses on the possibility of the controlling the mind through breathing.

The mind is the interpreter of the five senses, and therefore controls everything we experience. A strong mind makes a person reach great heights in life. A weak minded person's life is as weak as his/her mind. Your life is how the mind is. You are how the mind is. Therefore, mind is the master of the self, and the king of the country within. That is why a king in the Tamil language is called mannan. The mind is called manam. The one who can conquer his own mind is called the mannan, and he is the one who can stand the test of time. Our senses change over time, our thoughts and actions change over time, and they may even cease to exist as we age, but our mind lingers with us for entire life. Therefore, mind is the leader of the town.

The horse he (the mind) climbs on towards liberation – this horse is a symbolic representation of our breathing or pranan (prana), the vital energy that flows inside us because of the breathing process. Breathing is referred to as the horse that our leader, the mind clings onto. One might question why should the mind cling onto the breathing and not to the senses? Because a mind that goes after senses is an outward journey - a journey filled with sufferings and emotional attachments. Therefore, a mind requires a medium (horse) that goes inward. This inward journey is aimed towards liberation. Therefore the mind, the wise head of the town, chooses a path to liberation and clings on to the breathing. Because mind is a powerful tool for our liberation and happiness, but not for indulging in sufferings, it makes perfect sense why Thirumoolar suggests to use the horse of breathing rather than those five powerful senses for its inner exploration.

The word matru (other) in the second line has a deeper meaning as follows. It means that the breathing is one of the more than one horses that the mind uses. We know that there are five kottam (layers or kosha) that make us as we discussed earlier, and mind is one of them. Pranamaya kottam is between mind and body. That tells us that breathing can bind mind and body together. The horse that mind uses is breathing. But the word 'other' indicates that a breathe is just another horse that mind employs. That means mind employs several horses, or more than one horses at least. For instance, among the five kottam, mind can use pranamaya kottam on one side or vignanamaya kottam (wisdom layer) on the other side. By regulating the breathing one could facilitate the mind to transcend to the next inner layer, which Thirumoolar denotes as the other horse that mind could ride.

It will heed to truthful ones – Yes, the horse (the breathing) may look subtle, gentle, but it will respond genuinely to those who practise truthfully. A curious mind will then ask, "What is being truthful here and who are the truthful practitioners?" Here comes the reason why many of the yoga texts are cryptic in nature, not revealing completely what it is all about. That is one stage of stopping it from getting to the wrong hands. That is, we hear mythical stories of demons getting enormous power from the God by ardent penance. However, later they use it against God, or other creations. Therefore, Thirumoolar cautions here that these practices or the horse of breathing will respond only to those who practices with good intention.

The untruthful, gets toppled – To those who are entering into the practice for an untruthful cause, bad intention, and the horse will not respond and can even topple. A right mindset is a prerequisite here. It could also mean that if you practice sincerely, with diligence, the horse will obey you. If not, the horse will topple you. Thus the first poem outlines us the importance of breathing and how it relates to mind, five senses, and then sets the stage for the practice of pranayamam.

Practice:

How do we practice to put our mind on to the horse of breathing? You could follow breathing if you already learned the technique of listening to the breathing. Now be aware that the mind is constantly wandering. For those who could use some additional help following are some easy steps:

Choose a comfortable seating. In the beginning a calm place is good. As you become experienced, no external sound would bother you much. Therefore, begin with choosing a calm place and a comfortable seating. Close your eyes and position the mind in the middle of your forehead. Or you can think of the throat, or you can put the mind on the tip of the nostril. Now, you don't have to do any special exercise to the breathing. Just breath normally. It can be a slow deep breath, or shallow or mixed any way as your body demands; or in any way as it occurs naturally. Now you will watch the breathing going in and out from the spot where you chose, the forehead, throat, or tip of the nostril etc. The mind follows breathing either by standing in one of these places or moving with the forefront of breathing. If for any reason you are uncomfortable, stop the exercise and do normal breathing.

It may be good to practice this initially for 10-15 minutes. Beginning with a shorter time and increasing it slowly is always a good idea when it comes to breathing exercises. Also, early mornings and the evening times are good times to practice. One can perform pranayamam even during commutes as well.

Benefits of watching the breathing:

Normally we do not pay attention to our breathing process. As a result, the breathing tends to become fast and shallow. Once we start to watch, the breathing also calms down, just like an unruly kid tamed by the elders' watch. Let's say, our normal breathing rate is about 15 times per minute, the breath awareness reduces the number to 10 or even lower per minute. A research study suggests that slowing down the breathing to 7 times per minute is highly beneficial to hypertensive patients. Slow breathing relaxes the body, chest muscles, promotes abdominal breathing, activates stronger diaphragmatic movements, and as a result stimulates the vagal nerves. The net result? pranayamam keeps you more relaxed, a physical benefit. The intangible benefits including, a calm mind and a refreshed soul. A regular practice of pranayamam make one's life better and helps staying away from negative and toxic energy. Therefore focusing on breathing is a good practice to control the mind.

CHAPTER 2
CONTROL THE TWO HORSES

Original Version (Tamil)

ஆரியன் நல்லன் குதிரை இரண்டுள
வீசிப் பிடிக்கும் விரகறிவாரில்லை
கூரிய நாதன் குருவின் அருள் பெற்றால்
வாரிப் பிடிக்க வசப்படும் தானே

Transliteration

Ariyan nallan kudhirai irandula

Veesip pidikkum virakarivarillai

Kooriya naadhan kuruvin arul petral

Vaarip pidikka vasappadum thaane.

Translation

The good pranan has two horses

People don't know how to catch/tame the two horses

If one gets the grace of a benevolent Guru

Then the two horses will obey.

Pranan is the force of life flowing within all of us. This is the life energy that drives all living beings. pranan is present in both one-cell organisms, as well as multicellular organisms. It is not just breathing. It is not oxygen. It is the force or Sakthi that keeps us alive.

A bacterium may not require oxygen to survive (so does a plant), but they both have pranan or life. Different organisms manifest different forms of pranan. For example, in humans it is through the two nostrils (Naasi in Tamil): left nostril (idakalai or ida naadi) and the right nostril (pingalai or pingala naadi). The left is also referred as Chandra naadi (means moon), which signifies feminine and calming. The right is also referred as Soorya naadi (means sun), which is warm and masculine. Circulation of the air through these nostrils is important for life. In reality, our nasal cycle alternates the breathing from one nostril to the other every about 2 hours throughout the day. This alternation of the nasal cycle has been cited in the modern literature/medicine as a mechanism to avoid drying of the airway if it were to be flowing constantly through both nostrils. As a Scientist, this makes perfect sense to me.

In addition, there are several other functions of the alternation of the breathing cycle. For instance, if breathing through the right nostril is dominant, it creates a warmth sensation, and a rise in the activity of the left brain, whereas the opposite is true for the left nostril. The dominance of the right brain leads to activities such as imagination, creativity, daydreaming, motor skills, intuition, paying more attention to the tune of the song rather than the words, and looking at the holistic picture rather than details. On the contrary, the activation of the left brain is associated with activities such as logic, mathematics, analysis, computation, words, and linear thinking. As the activation of both left and right brain is important for a balanced life, it can be inferred that the alternation of the nasal breathing pattern regulates key brain functions.

Another key aspect of alternation of left and right breathing is their link to the sympathetic and parasympathetic nervous systems (both are parts of the autonomous nervous system). The sympathetic nervous system is linked to the fight or flight response or the stress response. Activation of sympathetic nervous system is important and necessary to cope up with acute stressful situations. During this time the sympathetic nervous system stimulates hormones such as adrenaline, epinephrine, norepinephrine that activate the survival mechanisms, promotes faster heart beat, increased sugar availability for the muscles, facilitating higher physical activity/energy level that all are necessary to combat the emergency situation. On the other hand, the parasympathetic system is involved in relaxation response or the "rest-and-digest" response. It activates the vagal and other nerves that promote activities such as salivation, lacrimation, urination, digestion, and defecation. As this is a relaxation response, naturally the amount of hormones associated with stress are reduced and those that promote our immune functions, and learning and memory are elevated. Activation of sympathetic and parasympathetic nervous systems in a balanced manner is a sign of healthy physical and mental status.

It may be possible that the alterations in the brain response due to alternative breathing cycle could be that the air is focused on distinctive nerve centers that subsequently stimulate the right and left brain response. Either it is the focus point of the airflow inside the nostrils or the outside of the nostrils could be activated differently. Let me explain this in detail. The outside of each nostril has a little dimple and an elevation. This is the part where people wear nose stud. This spot is a nerve and circulatory junction or plexus. Modern anatomy identifies the circulatory plexus as Kiesselbach's plexus. These two nostril plexus are a part of the ten naadi (nerve plexus) that are key to our function. The ten naadi are Ida, Pingala, Suzhumunai, Siguvai, Purudan, Kanthari, Athi, Alambudai, Sangini, and Kuhu. Of these Ida (left nostril) and Pingalai (right nostril) are located in the respective nostrils. During dominant activation of each nostril it may be that the nerves in that part of the nostril are activated more than the other nostril. This may not be felt with the movement of the nostrils, as it may be too subtle. But the activation of these nerves could be measured to find out how they are different when each side is activated. These nostril nerves are connected to the opposite sides of the brain hemispheres. The nerves that are found in the lower part of the face (nostrils, mouth, and ears) are controlled by the opposite hemispheres (contralateral) whereas nerves that control the upper part of the face (eyes, and forehead) are from the both sides of the hemisphere. It could therefore be understood that the left nostril nerves are connected to the right hemisphere and vice versa. It has to be borne in mind that brain hemispheres are not working as separate entities but rather work together. Another way how breathing through individual nostrils can influence separate parts of the brain could be that other structures such as the nasal capillaries, and sinuses located on each nasal pathway could allow gas exchange, just like what happens in the alveoli or the air sacs of the lungs, but to a much lesser extent. The availability of oxygen in these sinuses and capillaries could lead to secretion into the nearby blood flow (internal carotid artery for example) which then directly influences flow to that part of the brain.

Now let us take a look at the poem. The one who resides in this body is a good person. This first line establishes the basic truth about our SELF. We may think that we are corrupt, impure and while determining or analyzing who we are, all the not-so-good qualities come to the surface and remind us that we are not suitable to be called as 'good.' However, yoga philosophy as much as it talks about the transience (nilayamai), it always reminds us that we are part of the universal truth, the perfect being. We may be covered by layers of external impurities, but deep down we are the pure ones. Yoga is mainly about removing these external layers and ideas, and gets to realize the true self and be one with that. That is the reason Thirumoolar says that we are good; the self is good as a positive affirmation to begin this song.

The next words say that this Good person has two horses. Two horses are the two nostrils as we saw before. He uses the term horses, to represent again that our breathing can be as wild as a horse, but also as controllable as horses. Remember his reference to the process of breathing as horse in his very first song on pranayamam. This reference creates a picture in our mind about the nature of breathing while it is autonomous function, it can be voluntarily regulated and controlled to our benefit.

The second line says, "People don't know how to catch/tame the two horses"

In many of his poems, Thirumoolar uses a negative connotation first, that there is none who does it. Later he would come back and say if you know that then you are going to be a great one. This is a way of teaching the young ones as well. For a new, fresh mind, a word like this will go a long way. Most of the times when I teach my kids, I use this strategy. "Think, there is nobody in your class, pod, school who could possibly know this yoga technique!" This method of teaching, while makes them think they are doing something weird and crazy, they also get a positive attitude developed towards their new skill. Who knows one day schools may have a yoga class, and I have to come up with something else to challenge! Thirumoolar says nobody knows the technique of catching the horse. He uses words that would make us picturize someone with a lasso to get the horse. The term viragu also is to do with skills and determination/courage.

The third line
கூரிய நாதன் குருவின் அருள் பெற்றால்
If you get the compassion/grace of the Guru who is sharp –

There could be several masters, but find the one who has demonstrated expertise in the field of breathing. Gain his compassion, be his sincere disciple so his grace is upon you. In the Siddha system, the teachings are not always open, not a lecture type in front of all the students. At least not all of the teachings. The Guru chooses a certain type of student to teach a specific skill. This depends upon the Guru's ability to closely observe the disciple and evaluate his or her ability to learn that skill. Only if the Guru trusts you and be comfortable with you, you can get to learn it. This is an indirect way to tell us to do our best as students. This line also could mean us to identify the Guru within and follow. There may be external Guru only for the first few steps. After those first initiation, everyone must follow his or her own master within. This is a great combination of two lights clearing our way.

The fourth line

வாரிப் பிடிக்க வசப்படும் தானே.

If you catch (those horses) they will be yours.

The two horses are yours when you get hold of them. They cannot run away. The breathing will obey you. We feel that nothing is under our control at times. There may be things going on with our physical state, mental state, and relationships. Our power to control the issue of not being able to iron out an issue with a friend does not seem to be in our control. We get into arguments. We try to help by providing assistance and advice. Things do not seem to work. We feel it is not in our control any more. The situation is out of our hands. Pain is another great example. The pain that is caused by various diseases targets our sole determination. Our ability to tolerate and withstand is greatly reduced. When in pain we pay heed to the pain. We become the subordinates of the pain and look for a different master, the medication. Though medications help, the pain doesn't always listen to oxycodone or at least not in the same dose. You keep on increasing it and taking them more frequently. Breathing regulation might do wonders in chronic pain patients.

Another way to look at the Tamil word vaari used in the fourth line is it refers to a passage. Although this word is used to denote water, there could be broader interpretations. If one catches the passage, then the two horses will obey/heed to you. Focusing on the passage i.e. the respiratory pathway will divert your attention towards just breathing. Mind is in-sync with breath at this stage. When you inhale and exhale you watch how breathing goes in and out. Even the small waves, the curves that are created by the air waves can be felt when one can focus on the breathing by placing their mind on breathing. Our mind when away from the breathing has places to wander about. Its worries, anxiousness, problems of the present, past and future, all can occupy the mind. However, a mind that is stationed on breathing is anchored.

Practice:

The practice for this poem could be same as that of the first one, listening to the breathing process and trying to understand that we can regulate how we breathe.

CHAPTER 3
HAPPINESS FROM WITHIN

Original Version (Tamil)
புள்ளினும் மிக்க புரவியைக் கைக்கொண்டால்
கள்ளுண்ண வேண்டாம் தானே களிதரும்
துள்ளி நடப்பிக்கும் சோம்பு தவிர்ப்பிக்கும்
உள்ளது சொன்னோம் உணர்வுடையோர்க்கே

Transliteration
Pullinum mikka puraviyaik kaikkondaal
Kallunna vendaam thaane kali tharum
Thulli nadappikkum sombu thavirpikkum
Ulladhu sonnom unarvudai yorke.

Translation
Learning how to ride the horse that is faster than a bird
You do not need wine; the breath will give you the joy
You'll be energetic; no more idleness
I say this to those who are conscious.

We all would like to be happy for ever. We find happiness in several things around us. Happiness flows into us from friendship, love, sharing, comfort, and materials. When such external factors are withdrawn it is not easy for us to be happy. Is there a way we could find joy from within our own selves? Thirumoolar says "Yes!" in this chapter.

This happened sometimes around 2012. I went to India to celebrate Pongal (a popular harvest festival celebrated in Tamilnadu and other parts of India). I witnessed one of my younger cousins, in early 20s, lying in the middle of the road due to intoxication. I learnt a little later that he took-up this drinking habit as early as 17. It was very shocking to see a young, beautiful mind getting destroyed by illicit habits. The fellow citizens of my hometown reprimanded this lad to behave himself in public places. We used to be great buddies (despite our age differences), but his indulgence in drinking created some distance between us. I decided to fix this. One early morning I met his parents to probe more on how he derailed himself. As a way-out, I suggested yoga and even offered to help him get started with it. They were indeed happy, afterall he was their only son. My uncle who once felt helpless suddenly saw a ray of light in his life. Because he is known and respected for his benevolence and devotion to God, he very much wanted the same for his son.

I asked my cousin to come to our terrace the next morning where we hold yoga classes. The terrace is surrounded by a moringa, narathai (type of lemon/orange), nelli, mango and coconut trees. There is no roof or tall walls. The sky was clear and open above us. There were some clouds on the eastern side, just enough to block the morning son. I started off with surya vanakkam (sun salutation; to reconnect his body with his mind and spirit). To my surprise, he embraced it very quick even though I could see his arms, legs and whole body trembling while performing this exercise. I encouraged him and appreciated his dedication. Subsequently, I introduced breathing exercises. He did quite well but he was a reverse breather (i.e., tummy goes in during inhale). However, this can be fixed. The first session ended, but he was too curious to have the next one. In my own experience, as other teachers would agree as well, pranayamam can provide immense benefits if it is performed during the early hours of the day. The next day, at 5.40 am I heard him knocking my door. Clearly, the lad was getting an A grade for effort! I am so happy that he is committed to change his habit and his way of life. It makes me think that everyone needs someone to mentor them and help back in track in the event of derailment. Harsh words or reprimand hardly wins (in my opinion!). The news of unlocking one's one value through early morning yoga spread across the street. I am pleasantly surprised to see many kids joining the bandwagon. They say a teacher grows only when the student grows and empowers the society. This was what I saw. The lad who was once an alcoholic, now turned into a disciplined yoga practitioner and a mentor to the other kids in the nighborhood. People listened to him. In my view, a good supportive system, and a caring mentor is all one needs to learn and grow during testing times. I learned later he is still a yoga practitioner and is working abroad in Saudi Arabia as a construction worker.

The episode made me ask questions such as "Why do we drink, when do we drink, how much do we drink? The need to drink arises upon biochemical changes in the brain. A person who has tasted alcohol and seen its hallucinogenic effects finds a temporary joy, and an opportunity to forget worries. For that person, this is a way to be happy. Being happy is the ultimate joy one can get. If we get it through a mere drink we feel that the drink is the key to happiness. We reach out to the drink whenever we want happiness, whenever we want to forget the past, present and future. In the Indian context, youth already think that they have less responsibility as long as their parents are alive and earning. Because the child grows up and lives with parents until or even after his/her marriage. This gives the youth the basic food and shelter security. Whatever they could earn, either as a white-collar job or a daily wage worker, they could use a considerable portion of it for their pleasure. These days unfortunately it is booze. The friendship is also unique to India. Often one friend pays for the whole group to purchase of food or drinks. When we go out to eat to eat with friends we do not order either our own individual dishes or eat our own dish. Everybody will be eating every single dish on the table. There is always this big chaos, excitement and boundless sharing, especially when drinking is involved. To enjoy the wonderful positive feelings, sharing, friendship and the joy, they resort to booze again and again, and soon get addicted.

Addiction is the activation of reward cycles in the brain. For example, in addicted individuals the biochemical changes occur in their body include, the increased production of endorphins, brain derived neurotrophic factor (BDNF), and other feel good hormones that help neurons grow and survive. These biochemicals have distinct effects on the specific regions of the brain. Recent studies have shown that protein molecules such as BDNF are expressed more as a result of addiction, for instance immediately after taking a puff or booze. Increased BDNF leads to a feeling of wellbeing. Those who are addicted may not be looking for another dose if they had enough BDNF or endorphin.

I got exposed to alcohol at the age of 26. Although I am not a regular drinker I have had episodes of binge drinking. Most of the experiences have been to be happy and make others in my company ultimately happy. Though I have said to myself that this is not a healthy habit I had been doing this often at some point of time. Interestingly, I have lived the life as a teetotaler as well. Every time I consume alcohol, it unleashes the fun and creative side of me; people make me sing as well and I experiment various singing styles/ragas.

Depending upon where I am, I dance too. Everything will appear relaxed, enjoyable; people appear more open and friendlier than before. I wouldn't mind being ridiculed if it is so. I am not opinionated. I am inclusive of all thoughts, characters and flavors. Alcohol has helped me to realize the existence of this vast space inside me that can accommodate differences as well. Alcohol showed me the great hall where everyone comes together to celebrate the festivities of life by signing, dancing and being cheerful. For this experience I resort to alcohol when I feel down, and in blues. Also, when I have tight moments, alcohol has been my companion. This may appear reasonable to relax with some external help. But what are the consequences of alcohol on my mind and body? The effect on body is obvious the next morning. The sickness lingers around from the morning till the evening. In and out I am sick the next day. Nothing would look positive or interesting. Long-term alcohol consumption is deleterious to several body functions. Effects of long-term alcohol on the brain are beyond the scope of this book; but studies show that brain cells die faster when we consume alcohol. Liver wears out quicker with alcohol. So what is the alternative?

Our body produces large number of chemicals. These could be proteins, small chains of amino acids called peptides, lipids, and carbohydrates. These biological molecules have profound effects on our mood. Endorphins, endocannabinoids have significant improvement on our mood and other brain functions. Anandamide is an endocannabionoid produced in our body. This is similar to cannabinoid from the plant Cannabis sativa (marijuana plant). Pot at low doses has a positive effects on mood, just like alcohol. But there is a negative side as well. With Anandamide our body has a limit, it cannot keep producing Anandamide without any control over it, unless there is some disease. I realized through experience that the best way to find solace and happiness is through yoga.

One of the best things that happened during my recent visit to India is the creation of yoga Education Trust. We envisioned that this organization would empower youth through yoga. We sensed that children would greatly benefit from this Trust, however adults with addiction and behavioral problems might equally find it helpful. Now the classes are being held at Bala Gurukulam, the home where I grew up. My father, a former middle school principal, committed his life for educating and empowering kids and the community. This instilled a thought in me to launch a formal primary school in the same village just for yoga; my mother intends to dedicate our ancestral home for this noble purpose. The early success we have had with the yoga classes up there convinces me that a yoga school will help educate and empower kids and adults.

The formation of yoga Education Trust became easier when I visited Ponnamaravathi where one of my close friends, Arivu Alangaram arranged a meeting for the interested members of a society who convene for reading Saiva Siddhantha at my friend's residence. Days before that visit Arivu had come to Thangamani's home where we had a get together with many friends. We all visited a local temple at my friend's native where we practiced pranayamam. It was a wonderful experience to be at the temple along with my childhood friends in a peaceful location at the temple's courtyard. Just in front of the Varadharaja Perumal statue we were sitting and practicing pranayamam. After that practice Arivu wanted me to visit his place. I told him about the idea of forming a charity organization for yoga. He took me to an auditor that is his family friend, and things moved quickly from there on.

For the classes at Bala Gurukulam, I gave the responsibility of conducting the classes to one of the students, my nephew, who also has had the habit of drinking alcohol. I am seeing that he takes the responsibility seriously and teaching the classes genuinely. He is also weaning off alcohol slowly. It may be possible that it is a synergistic combination of timing, company of the right people at the right place, plus the power of yoga itself. For my future research, I am planning to measure BDNF and other neurobiomarkers to look at their changes in addictive behavior before and after the yoga practice, especially pranayamam. Finally, it is my hypothesis that pranayamam by stimulating the same pathways that are activated by reward circuitry could reduce the addictive behaviors.

In sum, this poem outlines rather simple concept that can have a deep, meaningful impact on our lives: that is, if one controls the reins the material joys (example, alcohol) are unnecessary. The breath itself will create a sense of long-lasting excitement and happiness.

CHAPTER 4

THE POWER OF PRANAN

Original Version (Tamil)

பிராணன் மனத்தொடும் பேராது அடங்கிப்
பிராணன் இருக்கில் பிறப்பிறப்பில்லை
பிராணன் மடைமாறிப் பேச்சறுவித்துப்
பிராணன் அடைபேறு பெற்றுண்பீரே

Transliteration

Pranan manathodum peradhu adangi

Pranan irukkil pirapirappillai

Pranan madaimari pecharuvithu

Pranan adaiperu petrunpeere.

Translation

When pranan coalesces with the mind

Then there is no birth or death

By controlling the path of pranan

One could reap the ultimate benefits of it.

The term Pranan has a more extensive meaning than mere oxygen or the breath. It is the vital energy that is making life possible. When the external air that goes in, our vitality takes over it and flows as pranan. The word pranan is also called panan, which is derived from the word panam that means arrow. It is the pranan that flows throughout the body and holds the breath within the body. Pranan is the force that keeps us alive. We may be able to breathe without Pranan, as in assisted devices. Pranan is the link that connects mind and body. It is the second one of the five layers (Kottam). It is the one that could liberate us from the cycle of rebirths.

The ultimate destination of each soul is to finish the birth/death cycles. However, Thirumoolar believes in reincarnation theory. That is, our soul takes abode in different bodies during every birth. I always think that I could have been an underdeveloped or less evolved human in my last birth. Or I could have been a squirrel who knows. Many Sithars believed in reincarnation; it is adopted by Hindus in general. A classical poem by a great poetess, Avvaiyaar, signifies how hard it is to be born as humans (அரிதறிது மானிடர் ஆதல் அரிது). Even difficult would be to be born as a human without disabilities. Even without disabilities it is harder to be wise and educated. Even while wise and educated harder is to be charitable and do penance. If one is charitable and performs penance, then the heaven is wide open to them. This classical poem by Avvaiyaar manifest cultural belief prevailed in ancient Tamilnadu. Therefore the ultimate goal of human life is to use its fullest potential to elevate the soul so that it completes its life/birth cycle - a rebirth thus becomes unnecessary. This leads to a series of interesting questions: what happens if you are not born again? Where does the soul go or the Pranan goes to? The Pranan when leaves the body finds abode in celestial objects including the moon, the sun and the stars, Thirumoolar believes. In my view, pranan energy makes new stars and new planets. If the Pranan is not the disciplined kind, it does not reach the stars yet but rather hangs around to be reborn.

Some thoughts in the Sithar philosophy are that we have countless number of births of different or same kind. Therefore every soul or pranan has several chances to learn the techniques of avoiding the rebirth. Every birth is a great opportunity to evolve and be one with the soul or identify the bliss and to be content. If we stay at the level of any of the outer layers of five kottas (without reaching the bliss) in this birth there is a good chance we will be born again. That is why people adopt various techniques to avoid rebirth. These techniques could be devotion, services and wisdom (bhakti, karma, gnana yoga). It is the same life force that is functional in all the five kottas. Sometimes you are the body, and sometimes you are the mind. Yoga takes you through all of the layers and makes you realize you are one. The yoga way of life makes the soul content and blissful. The pranan when leaves the body will be good enough to reach the stars. There are several practices to elevate to this stage and, one of them is through the regulation of breathing.

In this poem Thirumoolar talks about the benefit of what happens if your pranan doesn't leave the mind, or if pranan clings on to the mind. Mind and breathe can easily be disconnected, as we often do. Our mind is engaged in hundreds of affairs each minute. It is not going to be still. Patanjali says preventing the amplification of the thoughts is yoga. Thirumoolar says latch the mind to the breathing. Once the mind is still with the breathing, then there is no birth or death. This also could mean that it is not literally birth and death; rather it is the cycles of momentary anabolism and catabolism of both mind and body. When the mind and pranan are still the metabolic rate goes down. There is stillness in the system. Slower the metabolic rate less the toxic waste produced in the body, and much less the deterioration of the system as a whole. So bring the mind and pranan together. If the pranan is with mind then there is no birth and death.

In the third line (பிராணன் மடைமாறிப் பேச்சறுவித்து) he says – change the flow of pranan from one kotta to the other in an evolutionarily increasing order, that is to move inwards. Don't just stay in body or pranan or mind or gnana, but rather move inwards to the bliss state. In the process of moving to the higher kottas you will attain stillness. It is the dynamic stillness or the silence. Thayumanavar, a saint says, "Lord, will my thirst be ever quenched unless I can head to the blissful ocean that cannot be explained with words (சொல்லில்

அடங்காச் சுகக்கடலில் வாய்மடுக்கின் அல்லால் என் தாகம் அறுமோ பராபரமே)." True, you cannot speak when your mind and pranan are together. What will you speak, and how could you speak? Let the pranan pass through through the kottas while you remain in silence. This is the ultimate goal of the soul. Attain the stage that pranan naturally has to attain.

It turns out that it is the body, and our mind that block the flow of pranan through normal development or evolution. We block it because of our ignorance like a kid blocking another at the doorstep, asking for the password to cross. The password is to let the pranan flow in with the mind to a higher level. Let the pranan cling to the mind. As we saw earlier, the easiest way to control mind is through putting it together with the Pranan. It is so close to us, but we do not appreciate it. Once we start looking at this it opens several other doors.

Lets revisit the word 'madai' in the third line. In agriculture, it is the technique to channelize water to different areas of the field. Basically we use the sand in the little waterways (called vaaikkal) to block one side and open the other so water can be diverted to other areas where it is needed - similar to blocking the vehicle traffic to open up railroad for the train to pass when needed. The Thayumanavar's quote that I mentioned above also uses the active verb 'vaay madukkil' meaning the place that water reaching the field. Vaay madai is the place where the water channel meets the field and enters into the crops. My thirst won't go away until and unless I reach the blissful state that I cannot describe with words – says Thayumanavar. It is interesting to note that these two saints both Thirumoolar and Thayumanavar use a similar idea. There are several such instances where great minds think alike. I used to think that 'madai maari' means attuning or altering the breathing between nostrils. Thirumoolar would have been technically explicit had he only wanted to specify alternate nostril breathing. Therefore, it is not the technique of doing alternate nostril breathing, it is the technique of moving the pranan to different kottas so pranan can attain the state of ultimate enlightenment also called nirvana.

CHAPTER 5

THE PRACTICE OF THIRUMOOLAR PRANAYAMAM

Original Version (Tamil)

ஏறுதல் பூரகம் ஈரெட்டு வாமத்தால்
ஆறுதல் அறுபத்து நாலதில் கும்பகம்
ஊறுதல் முப்பத்து ரெண்டதில் ரேசகம்
மாறுதல் ஒன்றின்கண் வஞ்சகம் ஆமே.

Transliteration

Erudhal poorakam iirettu vaamathaal

Aarudhal arubathu naaladhil kumbakam

Uurudhal muppathu rendadhil resakam

Maarudhal ondrinkan vanjakam aame.

Translation

Inhalation through left for sixteen maathirai is purakam

Holding inside for sixty-four maathirai is kumbakam

Exhalation for thirty-two maathirai is resakam

Know that the breath changes alternatively.

Before we get to understand the calculations specified in this Suthiram (Sutra/formula), one must get familiarized with the maathirai system in Tamil grammar. A maathirai is typically the length of time taken to blink the eyes, which is equivalent to the length of time to pronounce a short syllable. For example, in the word 'another' the time taken for you to spell the first 'a' would be one maathirai. Any short syllable approximating the length I just mentioned is one maathirai. Two maathirai will be the length of time we take to pronounce 'a' in the words for example 'apple' or 'automobile.' The 'a' sound in these two words is longer than the 'a' sound in 'another.' To put it simple, if the letter sounds short it is one maathirai, if the letter sounds long then it is 2 maathirai. The letters that are conjunctional/ending in nature, for example, the ending 'm' in "Mom" is a letter that sounds with a stop to it. The word 'symbol' has both an 'm' as a conjunct, and 'l' as the final stop. These letters sound for the length of half a maathirai time. Thus, based on the letters and their sounding length, the total number of maathirai for any given word could be calculated. For example, the word 'symbol' has

Sy - 1 maathirai

M - ½ maathirai

Bo - 1 maathirai

L - ½ maathirai

Total = 3 maathirai.

The length of time required to pronounce the word 'symbol' is therefore 3 maathirai. One can take any word and try to calculate the number of maathirai it will take to pronounce the word. However it must be acknowledged that the rules of calculating maathirai cannot be strictly applied to English words because of the varying pronunciation in English depending upon the word. But in Tamil, a letter is pronounced with the same length of time. All of the short syllables (குறில்/kuril) have one maathirai; all long syllables (நெடில்/nedil) have two maathirai and all conjunctures (ஒற்றெழுத்துக்கள்/ottrezhuthukkal) have half a maathirai (of course there are exceptions, but they are beyond the scope of this book!). To practice the pranayamam that Thirumoolar teaches in this verse it is not necessary for one to understand or know Tamil. I will give examples of words with specified lengths so you can either follow them or use something similar for your practice. The maathirai system is the ancient Tamil method to measure the timings and rhythm of words or phrases. This is found being used in dance, music and of course I find it to be used here in yoga. Thirumoolar adopted this method to specify the length of inhalation, exhalation and the holding of the breath in the exercise specified in this Suthiram.

Now lets see the messaging of the Suthiram. Inhale through the left nostril for 16 maathirai. He uses the phrase "ஈரெட்டு," which translates to "two times eight." Vamam means left nostril. For counting sixteen maathirai one could use the word "ஓம் நமசிவாய" ("Om Namasivaya"). The letters in 'om' is add up to two maathirai in total. So, Na = 1, ma = 1, si = 1, va = 2 (this is a long sounding 'a'); ya=1 plus "om" together amounts to 8 maathirai in total. So, for inhalation chant this word in your mind (not opening the mouth) two times. The number of times we repeat the chant is counted with fingers.

How to inhale through just the left nostril? I have seen people making faces trying to breath through one nostril! Before getting to the practice if you have a chance to see the online video please visit my website: PranaScience.com). Use the fingers in one hand (remember the other hand is counting the chants) for closing the nostril. The easiest way for most people and the suggested way is to use the thumb to close the right nostril (If you note I am using my right hand for this maneuver in the video on my website); the thumb is almost perpendicular to the ground or parallel to the nostril. The left nostril will be closed by using both little finger and ring finger together. This helps the complete closure of the nostrils (This step will be followed for exhalation in a later step given below).

Once the inhalation is complete, both the nostrils should be closed tightly so that no air escapes. This holding is for sixty four maathirai.

For this, one needs to chant the manthiram eight times. This is called kumbakam. Holding air helps us in many different ways as follows.

a. Kumbakam calms the chaotic waves in brain, meaning the unwanted noise in the nervous system is reduced and therefore sharpens the real signal or processes.

b. Breath-holding increases the amount of carbon dioxide present in the system because of breath holding. However as the carbon dioxide level is built up further (called hypercapnic), further production of carbon dioxide is reduced, oxygen consumption is also reduced. At this time the system learns to how to survive when the oxygen amount is low. This is especially beneficial when the system experiences low oxygen supply, say as in the case of an acute shortage of oxygen supply to the tissue (ischemic preconditioning). This is also a way to create a mild hypercapnic condition, which is beneficial in several conditions such as asthma.

c. It is shown that kumbakam synchronizes the neural circulatory and respiratory elements and thus allows the coordination of mind, body and breath.

d. Through research, we identified that inhalation after holding the breath releases a sudden outflow of saliva that contains several molecules of interest.

There is a personal anecdote to go with this poem. In January of 2005, I was visiting India to celebrate the harvest festival, Pongal. My father was still alive at that time. During that trip I purchased a book on Thirumanthiram at Palaniappa bookstore in Pudukkottai, Tamilnadu. I had seen the poems being quoted on the web, discussed in forums; I wanted to get a copy for myself and I did. When I was packing for my trip to America, one of my uncles jokingly asked me why I wanted to carry a book that weighs as much as two bricks; instead I could have packed eatables or curry powder that would last until the next year. Also he was amused if I could understand the ancient literary Tamil, which is usually convoluted. There is a common misconception among several people that the ancient Tamil literature is not easy to understand. While this is true in most cases, there are several literatures including Thirumanthiram can be read at ease without the use of a Tamil-to-Tamil dictionary. A quantum of patience is all takes to decipher the meaning. However, a prose or explanation text accompanying any book will make it very easy to understand. I found the text by Gna. Manickavasakan very helpful. Later I contacted the writer and appreciated him for his work; and years later I met him in person in Chennai. He is such a knowledgeable scholar who specializes in ancient Tamil literatures.

So, going back to 2005, I brought this book and started reading it. I was interested in the chapters on Attanga yoga including this chapter on pranayamam. I came across this poem number 568. Although the meaning of the original poem as explained by Gna. Manickavasakan matches with my thought process, he had not mentioned how to measure that while doing the practice. So I devised a method, coined a few phrases such as Om Namasivaya, Thamtha dheengina and Thomtha dheengina, the latter two are used in dance and music. I even published this in my blog in 2006 with a note that phrases like these were used to denote time, say in a dance. That was a wonderful feeling when I decoded a poem, and devised a method to practice it. I tried it. It was not easy at the beginning to count, breath, chant, close the eyes and coordinate all together and above all to watch inside. By practice it became easy. I started feeling different, fresh and brisk whenever I did this exercise. Soon this one became my routine. I do this at least 3-4 times in a week.

After moving back to MUSC from Yale by the end of 2006, I continued the practice. One day, I am not sure if it was 2010 or 2011, while I was doing my morning pranayamam, this exercise filled my mouth with saliva. I noticed it happens every time I practice pranayamam. I know saliva contains, in addition to digestive enzymes, several proteins, neurohormones and small peptides that could have multiple functions in our body. I recollected that in our childhood whenever we are stung by a bee or beetle or ant, or any scratch to the skin or wound the first thing we do is to apply our own saliva. It became apparent to me that this pranayamam practice induces saliva, and it should have proteins and other principles that could impact our mood, health and overall well being. I started researching further on salivary proteins, other stress hormones and small protein pieces or peptides. My biochemistry background was quite helpful in putting several complicated pieces into perspective. I came up with a long list of possible neurohormones that could be there in the saliva. I thought this will have an impact on neurodegenerative diseases - Alzheimer's disease (AD) and Sjogren's - and aging because saliva production is low in these disease conditions. I. I networked with eminent scientists/physicians who also work in MUSC. Two names must be mentioned here: first, Dr. Jacobo Mintzer, a globally acknowledged psychogeriatrician who conducts clinical trials in AD. Second, Dr. Graham Warren, a radiation oncologist and a strong proponent of smoking cessation.

Because of the novelty in my research ideas, I was able to get a positive nod from Dr. Mintzer. Through a brief discussion that happened in his black BMW and subsequent walk on his way to work, Dr. Mintzer was too enthused to transform the ideas on paper into meaningful science. I have the habit of pouring out all the keywords in the first few minutes during any conversation. I do this specifically to save others' precious time. This act works sometime, but sometimes it is (playfully) viewed as if I am hurrying things. In the case of Dr. Mintzer it actually worked more than what I wished for.

He listened to me patiently, asked several questions about yoga breathing during midway. When he heard the word nerve growth factor (NGF), he interjected me and asked whether I measure the NGF levels. After knowing that I did not tested the levels yet, he got curious and told me to prove it. While I am not sure whether Dr. Mintzer is a republican, he quoted ex-President Ronald Reagan's words aptly:" I trust you but I want to verify. "He was a great catalyst throughout my journey. I returned to the lab with a resolve to "Prove it." I have limited knowledge in clinical trials, but that did not stop me. With all the wonderful help from people at the South Carolina Clinical and Translational Research Institute (SCTR) my journey was pretty smooth. I got the approval from the Institutional Review Board (IRB) that reviews and approves all the research involving humans. I found a collaborating biostatistician, even got a small voucher support so I can give a $20 gift card to the participants and to buy reagents to measure the NGF level in the saliva samples that I would be collecting. The plan is to get 20 people, randomly assign them to two groups one would be doing 20 minutes of yoga breathing (consisting of two exercises, 10 minutes of Om Chanting, and 10 minutes of Thirumoolar pranayamam, TMP, discussed in this chapter), and the other group is called Attention Control. These ten Attention Control participants were reading a science article of their choice. All the participants from both the group were tested one on one with me. By the end of October 2013, I finished all the sample collection and completed the analysis in the following months.

The moment of truth has arrived. My analysis found that there was increased NGF levels in people who performed pranayamam compared to the control group. This was tested using two different biological techniques. While this is only a preliminary proof-of-the-concept study, I am positive that a large number of participants would still produce similar results. Our research work was readily accepted for publication in the widely respected journal - International Psychogeriatrics. This was one of the most memorable times in my life. Because I was feeling that I am filled with new ideas, brilliance, wonderful collaborators, and I could achieve what I planned. I started another set of analysis looking at fine changes in saliva before and after yoga breathing. For this I first used my own Pre and Post samples from 6 different days and gave them to Ms. Alison Bland, who worked with Dr. Mike Janech. Mike is another wonderful energetic collaborator who graciously offered his time and labv once he heard my idea. Initially he was a bit skeptical, but to his surprise he observed changes in saliva levels as a result of pranayamam. Using mass spectra, we monitored at least 22 different proteins that altered (some go up and some go down) their levels as a result of pranayamam. It was something that I had speculated, but got excited when I elucidated the relevant proteins. Some of the proteins that made me jump for joy were DMBT1, Kallikrein, CRISP3, and Immunoglobulins etc. For example, the levels of DMBT1 is greatly reduced in brain tumors. That is why it is called 'deleted in malignant brain tumors 1.' This protein is needed to protect us from cancer, but this is deleted in tumor cells as cancer thinks DMBT1 is a hindrance to their cancerous growth. Contrary to the cancer scenario, people from the test groups (yoga breathing group) had stimulated DMBT1 in their saliva. DMBT1 is found to be deleted not just in brain tumors, but also in other cancers such as breast, prostate and lung cancers. It is considered as a key biomarker (a signal that this is linked to a disease) in breast cancer. These findings were the subject of our second research paper that we published in the journal Evidence Based Complementary and Alternative Medicine. It is amazing to see how pranayamam practice changes the biochemical profile of human body, by increasing the production of saliva. Our analysis laid groundwork for further probe.

My initial interaction with Dr. Tanaka of University of Texas in Austin and subsequent collaboration with Dr. Stacy Hunter at Pure Action resulted in the form of a research grant to continue our research. Pure Action is a yoga research organization run by a wonderful couple Jeff and Mardi Chen and their energetic group of Yogis in Austin. Our study funded by Pure Action was to inspect inflammatory cytokine profile in the saliva. Our analysis provided interesting insights. We found that key cytokines, a class of proteins that mediate inflammation were found decreased after pranayamam. These results were published in another reputed scientific journal called BMC Complementary and Alternative Medicine. A subsequent research study to measure changes in lipid levels in saliva was funded by the Lipidomics Core facility at MUSC, thanks to Dr. Ogretmen's team for collaborating on this. This also put me in frontline for crowd funding by Donors Cure (which has not yet taken off as the organization is in the developing stage).

In the midst of all positive events, arrived a big blow. I was informed that the research support I enjoyed from the MUSC Cardiology division ended. I met with the Department Head and explained how my studies are truly first-of-its- kind, and a breakthrough approach to improve patient care. Nevertheless, there was not sufficient funds to support research in pranayamam. This is one of the unfortunate things for the researchers. Especially those who are first generation immigrants, it is becoming increasingly tedious to establish as independently funded investigators. That topic is beyond the scope of this book and I am not inclined to elaborate on this. Fortunately I had the contact of Dr. Graham Warren whom I listened to speaking in a symposium on smoking cessation. I had contacted him to explore to use yoga for smoking cessation. He liked the idea, and while discussing he came to know about my expertise in cell signaling and learnt about my position in Cardiology was going to end. He asked if I am interested in joining his team. I thought it was a fabulous idea, partly he is supportive of my yoga studies; even promised me a 20% time to work on yoga. I moved to Hollings Cancer Center in July 2014 where I continue to work with Graham on smoking/cancer/radiation therapy/genetic variation, and yoga of course.

Throughout the turbulent times in my professional life I had clinched tightly on to my yoga practice, especially pranayamam. It helped me gain my energy and vitality every time I have fallen. I love to be a smiling man, never want to be cunning, strict and grumpy or old. I think yoga is giving me exactly what I need. Pranayamam, in particular, still the prominent one in my practice and classes. You can see a video of me showing the practice at my website: www.PranaScience.com

Hope this exercise can give you the same or even more benefits than what I found.

CHAPTER 6

WITH BLESSINGS FROM THE GURU

Original Version (Tamil)

வளியினை வாங்கி வயத்தில் அடக்கில்
பளிங்கொத்துக் காயம் பழுக்கினும் பிஞ்சாம்
தெளியக் குருவின் திருவருள் பெற்றால்
வளியினும் வேட்டு அளியனும் ஆமே.

Transliteration

Valiyinai vaangi vayathil adakkil

Palingothu kaayam pazhukkinum pinjam

Theliyak kuruvin thiruvarul petral

Valiyinum vettu aliyanum aame.

Translation

If you could inhale and hold the breath

Even if your body is very aged, it will become young like marble.

If you receive the blessings of the benevolent teacher

Then you could win over the wind and become the one filled with love.

Holding the breath in general, like the one explained in Chapter 5, has several benefits. One of the searches the human civilization has partaken is to find a way to stay young forever. Longevity. Who would want to age, get ill, immobile, and sick, and then leave this body one day? How much fear we have in getting old? Let it be a character King Yayati in the Indian epic Mahabaratham where he would ask the youthfulness of his own son. Or, let it be the search for the fountain of youth, the search which is on for the youthfulness among civilizations of all ages. Recent studies show several molecular pathways that lead to the cellular aging process. Stress, inflammation, cellular death, oxidative damage, radiation damage, defective antioxidant status, and environmental and lifestyle factors – all could affect aging. There was a king in Tamilnadu named Athiyaman. He was very charitable to all that came to him, and compassionate towards artists and poets. He was a good friend of a poetess named Avvaiyaar. Once when Athiyaman found a rare type of Indian gooseberry (Nelli) that is known to promote longevity, he carefully plucked it and brought it to Avvaiyaar and gave it to her without saying it was special. He did this so Avvaiyaar will be living longer and would do great service to the Tamil language through her literary skills. Only after eating it Avvaiyaar realized it was not a normal gooseberry but something very special. It is this story - and of course the medicinal values of the fruit - that prompted my wife Janaki and I to name our beloved daughter, Nelli! On one side there are humans that are on to everything to be young forever, and on the other side there are ones that could donate the youthfulness to somebody else as a symbol of love, or love of language.

Modern science tries to understand how aging could be prevented, delayed or cured. Calorie restriction emerged as one of the central avenues. In a stomach that is filled with diluted food, such as porridge, there is less calorie intake overall. A study suggested that fruit flies that consumed diluted food had lived approximately 10% longer than their counterparts that consumed normal diet. Along the lines, Thirukkural confirms that any meal should be eaten only after digesting a previous meal; this assures longevity (அற்றால் அளவறிந்து உண்க, அஃதுடம்பு பெற்றான் நெடிது உய்க்குமாறு).

Clearly, we can make a connection here that with the tummy filled with food we won't be able to practice pranayamam effectively.

In this poem Thirumoolar says that if you inhale and keep it within your hold, then it will help with longevity. The word vayathil means body, and has an interesting colloquial meaning of tummy too. You will see the tummy bulges when you inhale completely. You can see how it goes up and down when infants sleep. Tummy is also called vayiru. Thirumoolar used the term vayathil – vayam is the body. It could also mean the world. In any case, if you hold the air after inhalation, it will lead to longevity. This could be a way for lower caloric intake as well. Relate to how you feel after a Asana or pranayamam session, you do not feel really hungry. When I am on day long fasting I do a lot of pranayamam exercises intermittently. Believe me, there is no hunger, and on top I do not feel I am tired.

When Jesus had to feed five thousand people up in the mountain, he made food for everyone from five breads and two fishes. This is a biblical story. There is no problem for me to believe in this story as it is. But here is another way to look at this. He knew that five breads and two fishes won't be enough to feed all the five thousand people. He is the same one that said 'do you think that I live on food' when Satan tried to seduce him with food during his fasting. He is the one that said that I will teach you how to fish rather than giving you the fish. So how can we reduce this story to just about food. It could very well be that this story refers to what Jesus' preaching about five senses could be used to reduce the hunger, how the two fishes, the two naadi (ida and pingala) could be used to quench the hunger. This is the significance of those numbers five and two from this story. It is probably through the practice of pranayamam and meditation that Jesus was able to fast for forty days in search of truth!

pranayamam could help us with restrict our calories intake and thus helps with longevity. Including calorie restriction, there could be several mechanisms how pranayamam could result in longevity. For instance:

1. Pranayamam could promote the mobilization of stem cells from within the bone marrow, and allow them to migrate and differentiate in tissues where a cell replacement or tissue regeneration is necessary. Studies show that low levels of oxygen (hypoxia) in fact promotes the migration of progenitor cells, or stem cell precursors, out of the bone marrow. Pranayamam with breath holding creates a brief hypoxia (deficient oxygen levels) as well as hypercapnia (higher carbon dioxide levels), the best combination for the traffic of cells in blood stream. This creates a possibility of stem cell progenitors to migrate out of the bone marrow and reach the target organs, facilitating tissue repair and regeneration.

2. Factors such as NGF could promote or extend the life of the cells, especially under stressful conditions that otherwise would kill such cells. This could be very important in the case of brain and heart cells that do not use cell division to replace dead cells, rather could use new cells migrating into the injured space and differentiating to repair that area. As you may recall, our studies show that after practicing Thirumoolar's pranayamam for 10 minutes, even the novice participant show increase in NGF levels. Not only NGF, several other neurotrophins (proteins that stimulate neurons' survival) and biomolecules that would reduce overall stress in cells and promote longer, healthier life at the cellular level are produced after pranayamam.

I want to mention one of my adventurous experiments in the year 2013. First, I collected saliva under four different conditions: 1) normal basal saliva that I collected just prior to the following exercises, 2) saliva collected after five minutes of chanting Om, 3) saliva collected after five minutes of Thirumoolar pranayamam, and 4) saliva collected after I stressed myself out by watching horrific pictures for five minutes (Caution! I watched some extremely disturbing images from google images under the search term "Eelam war crime pictures" showing pictures of Tamil civilians wounded and dead during the Sri Lankan civil war from nearly the 1980s until the war officially ended in 2009). Those images were horrific to anyone except to those who committed the crime. The saliva I collected from these above four conditions (basal saliva, Om saliva, pranayamam saliva, and stressed out saliva), I hypothesized, would contain factors that will greatly alter the ability of the cells to survive. Second, I treated the cells (I was using a macrophage cell line called "RAW 264.7 cells") with the saliva from the above four conditions and then watched the next day how the cells looked under microscope. My results of this exploratory experiment were: the cells treated with basal saliva were looking normal; those treated with Om chanting and TMP saliva looked much healthier and looking differentiated to become a specialized cell; and, in a striking contrast, when the cells were treated with stressed out saliva that was collected when I was watching those genocide images, I could clearly see how the cells looked sick, I mean, really sick, and ready to die. This is one of the experiments I still do not have the means to fully characterize what factors are keeping the cells healthy or which cellular signaling components in the cells got affected. This experiment provides preliminary evidence that death and aging arise due to stress, and pranayamam is an excellent way to reducing/eliminating this stress and increasing healthier life at the cellular level.

The other essential component this poem talks about is to get the compassion or blessings of an enlightened master who practices benevolence. Why one needs the blessings or wisdom or compassion of his master? The word arul (அருள்) is normally translated as compassion or blessing. However, I view this this as wisdom, or the invisible connection between one and its master. The letter 'a' ('அ' 'a' in the word arul) also could denote something that you cannot see. This can be roughly equated to the English word non, or the 'a' in contrasting words such as typical vs. atypical. A material treasure is referred as porul (பொருள் translating to material) in Tamil.

In contrast, the intangible treasure that can only be perceived is termed as arul. Also the Tamil word uru means a tangible structure that we can see/touch, and in contrast aru is something that does not have a shape or structure (intangible) and hence therefore cannot be seen. That is why people refer God as both uru and aru, meaning God can be both form/formless. The letter 'L' in the words arul and porul refer to the intensity or density of the matter. Urul, Arul, Surul, Porul, and Marul are examples of words ending with the L. In all these words the letter L refers to the finishing characterization of the items denoted by those words. Poru refers to mass. The material that has a mass is called as a porul. Uru refers to structure or shape. It is probably the most prominent shape that man made, the wheel, that is referred as urul, urulai in Tamil. Similarly, the one for spiraled or shrunk is suru/surul. Therefore, arul is a collective substance that does not have a structure or shape or mass. Arul is emanating from the Guru. As it is coming from Guru it is given a further adjective Thiru, means of nobility, greatness, and wealthy. It adds much more value and respect to arul. We always pray to God for Her/His Thiru arul (also called thiruvarul as combined as per Tamil grammar).

Now, where and how do we get this Thiruvarul? This is where the fourth layer of five sheaths (kottam, or kosha or layer) comes in. The fourth sheath is the Vignanamaya kottam. As we saw earlier the first layer Annamaya kottam is the body; the second layer pranamaya kottam is the breathing; the third layer Manomaya kottam is the mind; the fourth layer Vignanamaya kottam is the wisdom; and finally the fifth kottam is the Anandamaya kottam or the bliss. In order to transcend the body, to reach the mind we need a bridge called the breath. The mind can transcend to the higher order and higher consciousness to the Vignanamaya kottam. Mind can interact with the higher consciousness to receive or send information. This sharing can be with those having a similar wavelength or thought process or nobility. The collective wisdom or consciousness could also be referred to as Arul. It is omnipresent. Including just in our vicinity, around us.

What we need to do is to surpass our own barriers of body, breath and mind to reach it. It is like gaining an internet access by typing the correct password. The Vignanamaya kottam is now opened to you. I have had several such experiences during meditation. It is a stage just in between conscious watching and sleep or unconsciousness. This is the sleep that saints call sleepless sleep. We can attain this stage of consciousness, or be one with the master. We can receive the wisdom of the master when we cross the first three layers. This wisdom will teach you the techniques to win over the wind/air/breath. You will learn several techniques, you will realize more ways to control and regulate breathing and will further be able to give to others. You yourself will be able to become a Guru and teach others the techniques revealed to you. The word Aliyan in the poem translates to the one who gives, or the one who loves. Because love is giving after all! At this point of high sharing just like your Guru, you become an embodiment of love. The Vignanamaya kottam has the Arul of great masters. They are waiting for us to come and find them. Body, breath and mind are not barriers, they are the bridges or pathways. Let us use these wonderful tools and reach out to the arul.

In summary, inhale the air and hold it within, then you can be young. You can refer to the youthfulness as the one referring to the soul or the spirit or the consciousness, or just the body. If you are blessed with the wisdom of the master, then you can win over the breath and give your wisdom to others.

CHAPTER 7

BREATH-HOLDING MAKES YOU A MASTER

Original Version (Tamil)

எங்கே இருக்கினும் பூரி இடத்திலே
அங்கே அது செய்ய ஆக்கைக்கு அழிவில்லை
அங்கே பிடித்து அது விட்டளவும் செல்லச்
சங்கே குறிக்கத் தலைவனும் ஆமே.

Transliteration

Enge irukkinum poori idathile

Ange adhu seyya aakkaikku azhivillai

Ange pidithu adhu vittalavum sella

Sange kurikka thalaivanum aame.

Translation

Wherever you may be, practice purakam (inhale) through the left nostril.

If you do so, the body shall not perish

Hold your breath as you say 'ang' and release it measured

And focus on the throat, you shall become a master.

If one looks at the above Suthiram superficially, the real meaning cannot be understood. A deeper realization is possible with the help of other Sithar poems. For example poems from Sivavakiyar, Karuvurar, and Subramaniya Sithar have helped me to get a clearer picture.

We have seen the positive effects of Kumbakam (breath holding) in the previous chapters. Prior to Kumbakam one could breathe in (Purakam) through both left or right or both the nostrils, Thirumoolar says Purakam is better if done through the left nostril. This could be approached from different angles. One has to find the right time to do this exercise, i.e., to perform this purakam when the breath is dominant through the left nostril. Remember, nasal cycle is specified in Thirumanthiram. Let me quickly refresh your memory again: left nostril (Friday, Monday, Wednesday), right nostril (Saturday, Sunday, Tuesday), and on Thursdays it is on left nostril if the moon is in growing phase while right nostril if the moon is in receding phase. This pattern needs to be checked before sunrise on each day. If it is not going in the specified nostril then one has to learn how to switch it to the desired nostril. This can be achieved by taking direct lessons from a learned Guru.

The best time to practice pranayamam is when the breath is going through the left nostril. The reason for this can only be speculated in my capacity with the available information. When left nostril is active, it pitches on a specific spot on the left side of the nasal passage, and stimulates nerves in those places which eventually is connected to specific areas in the contralateral side of the brain. Likewise the right nostril is situated such that the air goes in while inhalation impinges on a different area than the one focused via the left nostril. Even though both the nostrils end their division at the pharynx, there should be a reason why we have two nostrils unlike a star-nosed mole which has only one nostril.

The other possibility is that the left and right nostrils have the ida and pingala naadi respectively. The nerve plexus on the left and right nostrils differ. When the air is predominantly passing through that nostril, the ida or pingala plexus are the ones stimulated more. If one can sense the slightest tilt of the head can result in hearing sounds differently, then we should be able to appreciate that air passes through one nostril could be sensed differently from the other. Let us consider for a moment how our brain senses music. The language and music are processed differently by the different hemispheres of our brain. The left hemisphere processes language (lyrics) whereas the right hemisphere processes music (rhythm). Interestingly, the left ear is connected to the right hemisphere and right ear is connected to the left hemisphere. Of course both the hemispheres have to work together normally through the connectivity of corpus callosum. But each hemisphere has a different way of processing the inputs. The same scenario could be applicable for the breathing too, because just like the hearing, our left and right nostrils are connected to the opposite sides (contralateral) of the brain. That is one of the reasons we could observe the change in hemisphere dominance as the nasal cycle switches.

It is a great practice to watch which nostril is active at any given time or activity during the day. Watch carefully how, when and if the breathing switches first. Then watch what activities change the nostril dominance, and what activity you are engaged in. Still further, watch how moods can switch the nostril dominance. It is a feedback loop. One feeds the other. One controls the other. When we are angry, aroused versus when we are calm. See which nostril is drawing and releasing more air. Check which nostril is sensing the movement of airflow. When one of my older sisters gets angry they all say her nostrils start to flare. The feeling of anger stimulates a physiological response to breathe heavily. It might be that anger is a self-defensive, fight or flight response mechanism, and producing hormones that will stimulate the metabolic activity of muscles needed for a physiological response involving the whole body. Our life is a long learning process, and realizing or understanding our mind and body in itself requires a considerable amount of time and effort. Working with something just under our nose may be easy to begin with!

What happens when the air flows through one nostril? Air is an activator of our senses. Cool air, when touches our skin or hot air blowing on our face can be normally distinguished. It is not just the temperature that we could feel, it is also the flow, the pressure of blowing air, and the speed in which air is flowing into a spot can all be felt by our cells. Remember the extreme power of airflow that you experience from the hand driers in those paper towel free, environment friendly restrooms. Air flow can be felt not just by skin cells, but also by the cells that line the mucosal membrane (did I tell you the Tamil word for nose is mooku; this is the root for the word mucosal. The Tamil word sali relates to the drainage of the mucosal/salivary system. Interestingly several Tamil words could be linked to modern medical terms!).

Now, back to the mucosal membrane – lets do a simple a practice, bring the shape your lips just like you say the English alphabet O, and then start inhaling through the mouth. You will see the cold air flowing through the lips and travels on the upper surface of the tongue and reaches all the way to the throat. Means the nerve cells on this air passage can sense the flow of air. Now, the cells in those spots can be activated differently to produce a secretion of mucosal fluid. Our nervous system both sends and receives information from each location of the body. It sends signals to move, activate, and relax specific spots. At the same time brain receives signals from these external organs too. Classical way of neurotransmission is through a neurotransmitter like acetylcholine that is released by one neuron and taken up by others and so on in a relay system within femtoseconds to transmit the signal. This happens for both to and from signals from the brain. There is another way of signaling that is through retrograde axonal transport mechanism. Several neurochemicals use this mechanism. This is a mechanism by which brain cells get their information about the tissues, surroundings, and peripheral organs. Brain cells although can produce all the proteins they need for their growth and survival, they do receive information and nutrients or factors from other areas of the body. These factors are key information about the external environment, source of nourishment, and also the messengers of stress and illness.

For instance, nerve growth factor and other neurotrophins can be transported to the brain where they can stimulate the growth and survival of neurons. Also they provide information to the brain that the environment or the activity of the organism is stimulating. Say a sweet smell, or music or food or a good companion. It is a reward to brain, so brain can promote such functions/activities. Habits form like this. You go for a walk with your family, or for a tea with a workplace friend, or go to do a workout, your brain knows that you are going to do it, and it is the time. When the time arrives for entering into your activity your system is ready with its senses. You touch and feel, let it be the air, your friend's hands or the screens and buttons of a treadmill. They all provide the signals. Those signals stimulate local cells. They work to secrete the factors and send them to the brain and the brain uses them. Brain is a master, like a royal king, he won't go work in the farm to enjoy his grapes. It is produced in the fine valleys and brought to the king. The king enjoys them and send the farmer with lot of gifts. The farmer goes back happily and keeps working hard, and tries harder to produce finer grapes next time. This is mutually rewarding. This is how the interaction between our brain and other sensory inputs could be related. Here it is the cells lining the mucosa, the nostrils, mouth, or the throat that produce factors that nourish the brain.

Now, if we breathe through left or right nostril makes a difference because they impinge on separate spots on two different nasal passage. As mentioned earlier it is the dominance of one hemisphere over the other in a specific activity but eventually the information and activities affect both the hemispheres. But certainly specific areas of the hemispheres get stimulated based on where the air touches. And remember, the speed, bulk flow and the temperature of air also matter. That is one of the reasons Thirumoolar says to use the left nostril for these exercises. It might be to stimulate the right brain that is more holistic, intuitive, emotional, and creative than the left hemisphere.

One needs to consider the role of sinuses connected to each of the left and right nostrils. The sinuses are important air spaces within the respiratory system connecting it with the nervous, circulatory and endocrine systems. The sinuses provide an empty space to vibrate the air when we speak. Sinuses do exchange gas. It is not just the alveoli in the lungs that exchange gas with the blood. Sinuses have capillaries that can exchange gas that comes through. Sinuses also can produce nitric oxide when we do humming or similar exercises that vibrate or stimulate the sinuses. Nitric oxide has a wide range of positive roles including anti-oxidant and neurotransmitter functions that are known to improve the functions of the brain. It can easily diffuse through cell membranes unlike many other neurotransmitters that would require a specific receptor. Several breathing exercises stimulate or cleanse the passage of air through the sinuses. When the air circulation improves then the toxic waste build up is reduced in those areas. Some sinuses such as the sphenoid sinuses are very close to the arteries that supply blood to the brain. It may be possible that molecules like nitric oxide that are produced in the sinuses or in the nearby endocrine organs could be readily transported into the bloodstream that goes to the brain. Now considering left and right nostril dominance, one side of the brain could be supplied with blood enriched in neurohormones due to the local activity on the way. It makes perfect sense, isn't it!

The other meaning for the word 'idathile' in the first line of this poem is "in the same place." Because the Tamil word "Idam" could mean the Left side, or Place. If we consider the poem does not indicate the left nostril, then it may be referring to the external place. Do wherever you are, whenever you remember to do the exercise, breathe in, fill yourself with air, hold it, and release. Whether you are driving in your car, or working on your computer, doesn't matter. Just do it wherever you are, right there in the same place.

In this Suthiram there is another intricacy that became visible after I read the other Sitars' songs I mentioned in the beginning of this chapter. That is related to the word 'Ang.' The pronunciation of Ang involves the base of the tongue touches the end of the soft palate. A deeper practice, or a persistent sound like 'annnnngggggggg,' just like the sound of a bell ring, rinnnnggggg! Or the sound of the blowing of the conch shell. The conch in Tamil is called Sangu. It also means neck or throat. There is a striking connectivity here among languages. Anyways, the sound Ang could be like a cork or seal to hold the breath after you inhale. This action is important in the coordination of various muscles within the throat as it is the place of breathing, swallowing and speech. The action of holding the tongue on the back so it abuts the throat stimulates lot of saliva. Chanting 'Ang' is one of the practices in Siddha literature. I have designed an exercise on Ang chanting just like the Gong meditation. This involves chanting Ang in multiple forms and coordinating with the breathing. I could make a video, but this exercise is best understood when learned in person.

"If you do that then body shall not perish." This is a strong statement.

Thirumoolar knows that the body is not permanent. He knows that all the bodies will perish one day. But the meaning of this line is that we won't die abruptly, rather we will live a long healthy life. We will not suffer from numerous diseases while we live in this body. The term 'aakkai' in Tamil generally means body. But it also indicates anything that makes, or produces. Our body is the creator of activities, and functions. It makes good and bad. It is the main instrument for all our actions (aakai or aakku in Tamil becomes 'act' and "action'). If the body is good and strong we can function efficiently. If the body is afflicted with diseases, then we won't be able to perform even simple tasks. Therefore it is important to keep the body strong and able so it can function in its fullest capacity, and with plenty of creativity. When we are creative we have a meaning for this life.

Thirumoolar says in another poem, if we spoil this body, we spoil the spirit, and we never can attain the real wisdom. Here, in this poem to keep the body strong and healthy for a long period he says pranayamam is the way. Of which, the breath holding is one of the key exercises as we saw. He also says to focus on the throat chakra. Sangu means throat in Tamil. When we focus on the throat as we practice these breathing exercises our mind is still, standing unmoved in one place, and is able to control the senses much better. Once the senses are under our control and channelized in proper direction, then it is not tough to achieve success in anything that we do.

Once we know how much to inhale, how long to hold and how long to release, the measures of it, then we can become the leader. The word leader could mean the master of our body and mind. Once we achieve winning over our own mind and body, then we can easily win over the others and become a leader in the community, institutions, world or whatever we aspire!

CHAPTER 8

KICK THE DEATH AWAY

Original Version (Tamil)

ஏற்றி இறக்கி இருகாலும் பூரிக்கும்
காற்றைப் பிடிக்கும் கணக்கறி வாளரில்லை
காற்றைப் பிடிக்கும் கணக்கறி வாளர்க்குக்
கூற்றை உதைக்கும் குறி அதுவாமே.

Transliteration

Etri irakki irukaalum poorikkum

Kaatrai pidikkum kanakkari vaalarillai

Kaatrai pidikkum kanakkari vaalarkku

Kootrai udhaikkum kuri adhuvaame.

Translation

The pranan fills us flowing through both the left and right naadi; there is not many that knows the measurements of how to inhale, hold and exhale; for those that know these measurements, it is the instrument to kick death away.

Being a scientist and a pranayamam instructor, I meet over hundred people every month (at least). When I converse with others and share my expertise I am consistently "Wowed upon." They feel very energetic to learn about the everyday benefits of pranayamam. To be honest, sharing the wealth of knowledge to others energizes me as much as it energizes them. I love seeing their faces, at-ease relaxed breathing and friendly smiles. I would argue that repeated breathing exercise instills a positive and friendly mindset in everyone. Most doctors advices us to take a deep breath, but we always tend to forget that! In my class, I ensure that everyone remembers to take a deep breath, to breathe mindfully, to be aware of the rate of breathing, to alternate between breathing cycles using both nostrils, and several other way of regulating the breathing from the over fifty different pranayamam techniques.

After all, mortals can only breath finite number of times during their lives. This is analogous to a banking game that kids play. The banker gives every player certain amount of the money and the overall goal of the game is to use the money wisely. Some tend to spend them quickly, whereas some are very conservative. The concept of yoga breathing is very similar. The faster we breathe, the faster we empty our pockets (not a good sign of living!). The slower the breath, not only we perfect the art of breathing regulation, and could explore pranayamam further, but the results lend itself to longevity and a satisfied life. Doesn't it look interesting? Let me dive even deeper. We breathe about 15 times in a minute. Mathematically speaking, that is 900 breaths per hour, 21600 breaths a day, 7,884,000 breaths in a year and 551, 880,000 breaths in 70 years! For the sake of simplicity, let's say we have only 550 million breaths allotted for us during our entire life. Even if we control our breaths to 5 breaths per minute - and that too only for 5 minutes in each hour - our overall breathing load would be reduced to 521 million breaths in 70 years. A 31-million savings in our "breathing" account! This, in theory, would prolong the life for another four years! On the other hand if we expend more breaths per minute, we tend to lose years! It is not just the number of years that adds to the life, it is the healthy life that is added. I strongly suggest you to slow down on breathing (it's never too late to do the right thing!). Our time is limited, but by engaging in pranayamam we can prolong it.

I often get the question how slow-breathing prolongs life. Let us focus on the concept calorie restriction again. There are several studies that show calories restriction can extend lifespan by at least 10%. This was tested in mice from different strains or genetic backgrounds - similar to different ethnicities as in humans - and in multiple research centers to be certain that the data is reproducible. The mice that mimicked restricted calorie intake lived longer without any defects in physiological functions of course with a comparatively balanced body weight than the ad libitum fed (unrestricted food supply) eating counterparts. The researchers identified a key protein pathway involving a protein called mTOR (mechanistic/mammalian target of rapamycin) that performs numerous functions in a cell. For example, this protein regulates the metabolism of a cell and as a result the tissue and the whole body. One important pathway that mTOR controls is the protein biosynthesis that makes new proteins in the body using the nutrients that are supplied through diet. More the nutrients, more will be the protein synthesis. Similar to light and dark cycles (circadian rhythm) in our body there is a starvation-feeding cycle that keeps the mTOR dependent protein biosynthetic pathway going up and down in cycles. When the body has limited source of nutrients – fed at limited amounts and only when needed, then the cycle is maintained well. If there is a constant feeding, then the cycle is swaying towards pro-synthetic pathway. The regulatory brakes are off. The machinery keeps on making more proteins in abundance. This leads to the accumulation of both desired (functional) and undesired (dysfunctional) proteins. Normally the dysfunctional proteins and aged proteins are cleared by the protein degradation system in the cells. However, since there is an overload of proteins, the degradation is also diminished and this affects the other associated metabolic pathways leading to overall stress and dysfunction of the system. It is conceivable from this how we overfeed ourselves and feel inactive/lazy/lethargic, both physically and mentally.

The change in metabolism can be achieved through elements other than food restriction, physical exercise being the most common.

Numerous studies and my personal experience accentuate this notion. Additional elements that alters/regulates metabolism are breathing and proper mindset. Let us see one example of how mind can change the metabolism. Say we have a chain of thought that arouses us, anger for instance, then our breathing gets stronger and that fuels the metabolism. Here the ignition is from the mind. The same mind when in a calm state, say your favorite quiet place, serene scenery where a baby rests in the lap of the mother, your mind and breathing are calm; not as heavy as in an aroused state. This calmness slows down the metabolism.

Regulating the breathing could function in a way similar to dietary restriction. Of course here we channel the mind to instruct us how to perform the exercises. Mind is a command center whereas breathing is where the actions take place. While inhaling, holding and releasing in the fashion discussed in the previous chapters (Chapter 5 for instance), one can achieve a slower pace of breathing and hence attain a slower metabolic rate. One may wonder how this might take place. We try to understand it using biomarkers that are expressed in saliva. As saliva is a clear index of quicker changes in physical and mental status we chose to investigate salivary biomarkers. One of the markers for elevated stress level is salivary amylase, an enzyme that breaks down dietary carbohydrates to glucose. Guess what happens when there is more amylase? An increased breakdown of complex sugars to release glucose, therefore a metabolic upregulation. This is where pranayamam could be more beneficial. By engaging in this yoga breathing, one can increase saliva, reduce the salivary amylase production and hence can control the metabolic upregulation by reducing the production of sugars. This might be a difficult important to understand, but it is critical for a healthy living.

It is important to consider that breathing regulation by pranayamam can be used to both accelerate and decelerate the metabolic rate. For instance, there are fast breathing techniques such as Bhastrika which stimulate the metabolic rate; whereas slow breathing exercises such as Sheetali can reduce the metabolic rate. Just like the term exercise could encompass walking, jogging, running, sprinting and marathon racing, the concept of pranayamam encompasses a variety of techniques with distinct outcomes: in some cases it slows down the metabolic rate, some cases it increases it. This brings an interesting question - why one needs fast pranayamam? When our system is lethargic and resists active life style, fast pranayamam can fix that. Say in the morning we want to stimulate the system with some burst of energy. Just like the engine that gulps more fuel when it starts up. Fast breathing technique is similar to this. To warm us up in the cold mornings. Once we are charged, just like the green energy engines, we burn less calories to maintain alertness at both physical and mental levels and by creating less stress to the system. Thus pranayamam influences positively in reducing stress via a regulated breathing pattern. Reduced stress is the key to a healthy and disease-free life, and this is what Thirumoolar means by kicking the death away. Therefore, learn the methods and calculations of correct breathing techniques and live longer!

CHAPTER 9

BLESSINGS FROM A POISON EATER

Original Version (Tamil)

மேல்கீழ் நடுப்பக்கம் மிக்குறப் பூரித்துப்
பாலாம் ரேசகத்தால் உட்பதி வித்து
மாலாகி உந்தியுள் கும்பித்து வாங்கவே
ஆலாலம் உண்டான் அருள்பெற லாமே.

Transliteration

Mel kizh naduppakkam mikkura poorithu

Paalaam resakathaal utpadhivithu

Maalahi undhiyul kumbithu vaangave

Aalaalam undaan arul peralaame.

Translation

Hold the breath until the lower, upper and middle chest are completely filled; as you exhale at the step of resakam, which nourishes us like milk, tuck in the three parts of the chest inwards until a time you really need breath, and then inhale filling the tummy – if one does this, then they can get the blessings of the Lord (Siva) who survived the most poisonous venom.

There is an ancient Indian fable. Like most other fables, this one also has two opposing central characters: Devars (Gods; smart and clever) and Asurars (Demons; physically strong, but not clever). Well, the story goes like this. Both the Devars and Asurars embarked on a journey to churn out the nectar of immortal life (amudham) from an ocean that is filled with milk, a.k.a the cosmic ocean. This was more of a Devars' plan, but because of the physically demanding nature of the exercise the Asurars were tricked-in to join. The mighty Asurars used a huge mountain (Mandhira malai) as a churning pole and a serpent king (Vasuki) for their churning-string. As they churned, a terrible poison came out from the ocean and it started to blanket the universe. Completely clueless about their next step, as well as to save their lives and the universe from the venom, both the groups sought the help of Lord Siva. After acknowledging the situation, the venom was swallowed by Siva. However, because he ingested the venom the poison started to descend into his gut but stopped in the throat, thanks to Parvati (Siva's wife). Once their safety was assured, the two groups continued with the churning and surprised themselves with various gifts including the Goddess of wealth, a mighty elephant, a sacred cow, and a tree that grants wishes, a horse and finally the nectar. The story goes on, but in short the Devars used their wit and intelligence to save the nectar of immortal life from the Asurars whom they fear might use it for destructive purposes. As always, the might of the Asurars was outwitted by the cleverness of Devars.

Some think that Asurars were always cheated by Devars while others believe that to achieve your goals you should employ every possible strategies and tactics.

The purpose here is not to narrate a mythological story, but to bring its relevance to the present poem in pranayamam. At least, this is how I interpret it. By channeling the breath (serpent-king Vasuki) through the nostrils using brain or mind (churning-pole Mandhira malai) on one's own body or mooladhara chakkaram (ocean of milk), one can churn out longevity (nectar of immortal life).

Mooladhara chakram is believed to be the abode where life begins. Scientific research offers clue that we still have some reserve of early pluripotent stem cell population (cells that have the capability to give rise to different cell types) waiting for a stimulation. In addition, it offers hope that there are circulating stem cells all over our body; in almost all organs there are some resident stem cells (an undifferentiated cell that has the capability to develop into any cell type) too! The major source for these stem cells is mooladharam (located at the sacral plexus). As the name suggests, moolam means the source or origin, and aadharam means support or proof. Thus, we can interpret that the mooladharam as the place where the source of our body is preserved. Interestingly, mooladharam is often associated with Lord Ganesha because of his placement in the entrance of all temples.

The life source does not function on its own. It needs stimulation, exercise, nourishment or power to work. The butter is held within the cream; however, a churning process is required to bring it out. Similarly, the mooladharam is the source for life, happiness, bliss and youthfulness. It has the source cells that have the capability to repair damaged cells to keep the organs function ceaselessly during lifetime, and offers lifetime maintenance and warranty to our body. However, it demands regular premium. One need to pay to buy that warranty as it is not free. Similarly, to churn and stimulate mooladharam, one might use breath as the currency. One of the ways to stimulate mooladharam is explained in this poem by Thirumoolar.

During the normal inhalation process, we hardly pay attention to how we breathe. We think it happens on its own and we are mere passive bystanders. As a result, we end up breathing with our chest, or with the upper chamber. Chest breathing is not deep as it does not engage the diaphragm fully. It does not fill the full capacity of the lungs. Unless wet engage lungs to its full capacity, we are wasting its utility. In fact, slogans like "Use it or lose it" and "Motion is lotion" fit very well for the lungs. The tiny room in the lungs that do not get circulated by good air often could face more stress and as a result becomes more susceptible to diseases. Unless we watch how we breathe, the air circulation through the minute air sacs in the lungs is less efficient. Watching the breathing pattern for 24 hours is nearly impractical, however one can at least engage in this endeavor during the times of stress and fix it with supplying voluminous air circulation. This is what Thirumoolar means to fill the upper, lower and middle areas (of the chest/abdomen).

One might think filling-up the lungs with air is similar to filling-up the gas tank with petrol - there's a stopping point in near sight. But you will be surprised to see that it is a bottomless tank! You can forever fill-in more air even after reaching the threshold. Great yoga masters (for example, Swami Satchidananda) continuously preach to 'breath in little more.' This is what is reflected in Thirumoolar's writing as well. The word "Mikkura" used in the first line of this poem may refer to fullest, in excess, or a lot. Let us engage in filling-up our lungs to its full capacity, whenever possible. Many pranayamam exercises such as Bhastrika, alternate nostril breathing and of course Thirumoolar pranayamam (TMP) are great exercises where one can practice and experience the complete filling of the lungs.

Let's say the inhalation is done to its fullest capacity Thirumoolar now turn towards correcting the exhalation pattern. He preaches to tuck the tummy in as you practice the exhalation (resakam). And he uses a word Paalaam" which refers to milk that it will lead to. This can be understood as the exhalation process is able to stimulate nourishing factors just like milk. A curious mind will wonder how. Once you complete exhalation, after you inhale, there would be noticeable salivary production. Saliva is just an external indicator; it does not project completely what happens inside. Apart from the salivary glands there are numerous other glands in the body that are closely associated with the central nervous system. As the muscles of the diaphragm are stretched and contracted, the nerve plexus in the chest and abdominal area (the sacral, pelvis, and solar plexus referring to mooladharam, swadhittananm and manipuraka chakkaram respectively) are stimulated or stretched during exhalation. This leads to the activation of glands associated with those nerve centers. These glands produce factors locally and also some of them could be expressed systemically and available to other parts of the body via the blood circulation. To those regions where blood cannot reach on its own, they are transported via neurons, just like the NGF transported to the brain via retrograde axonal transport. The factors that revitalize all the body parts energize us to function better and boost our morale – all just like milk! That is the reason why Thirumoolar refers to resakam as milk. The good thing is all this happens without the problem of adding more calories or burping.

Now let us consider the third line of the poem. It talks about the re-inhalation. This line refers to a word maalaahi. This means a state of hallucination, delirium, or in Tamil mayakkam. Similar to a baby oscillating between sleep and awake states. The word 'maal' has meanings like the junction of light and dark (as in the evening). It refers to the state of a youth who sees a girl and wonders or hallucinates if she is an angel or someone who is as beautiful as a peacock as nicely described in Thirukkural (anangukol அணங்குகொல்). This is the current state of our being at the completion of resakam, right before we begin the next pranayamam cycle. This is the state we are nourished with the after-effects of a rewarding pranayamam cycle (similar to drinking milk). As you begin subsequent inhalation, ensure filling the abdomen and then proceed to filling the upper-chest chambers as stated above.

The word kumbi not necessarily refers only the abdomen, but also the entire thorax and abdominal area. Usually, only after a sound meal there is a sense of completeness in the abdomen region. However, the same feeling of fullness can be felt through inhalation as well. Whenever possible, many Saints suggest air (through deep inhalation) in the place of food. If beneficial effects can be achieved via breathing, shouldn't food intake be minimized? The green energy engine, our body, can use air as energy source rather than food. Of course you need some fuel (either electricity or gas) to start the engine, as well as to store the solar energy. Similarly, you need food to preserve the vital functions, but the other factors can be produced as a consequence of disciplined breathing. Neither food nor supplements can achieve what a regulated, yoga breathing can.

By engaging in the pranayamam cycle, in a disciplined fashion, one has the blessings of Lord Siva to live longer. As stated earlier, Lord Siva ingested a terrible poison that emanated during the churning process. Poison, perceived deadly during most circumstances, can be beneficial in small amounts. The venom inadvertently produced in the process of cultivating ourselves through pranayamam could also be our big ego. Let our awareness, the Siva that dwells within us, ingest it and save the whole process. Similarly, everything produced during the churning process could be a symbol of the benefits we could get from the pranayamam practice.

Thus, a defined focus on inhaling air, holding and subsequently exhaling it can have a profound impact on our everyday wellbeing.

CHAPTER 10

WHEN A CHANT BECOMES THE BREATH

Original Version (Tamil)

வாமத்தால் ஈரெட்டு மாத்திரை பூரித்தே
ஏமுற்ற முப்பத்தி ரெண்டும் இரேசித்துக்
காமுற்ற பிங்கலைக் கண்ணாக இவ்விரண்டு
ஓமத்தால் எட்டெட்டுக் கும்பிக்க உண்மையே!

Transliteration

Vaamathaal eerettu maathirai poorithe

Emutra muppathi rendum resithu

Kaamutra pingalai kannaaha ivvirandu

Oomathaal ettettu kumbikka unmaiye.

Translation

Inhale through left nostril for sixteen maathirai

Exhale for thirty two maathirai through right nostril

Hold the breath for sixty four maathirai

Let the truth be revealed.

The meaning of this Suthiram (formula), in essence, is similar to the poem discussed in chapter 5 (Suthiram 568). Some might find this redundant. Back in the days, palm-leaf manuscript was the preferred choice for authors (obviously, paper was not discovered then). These leaves were extensively processed to test the suitability and durability, and poems were written on them using iron stylus (called ezhuthaani). These palm leaf manuscripts are referred as olai suvadi in Tamil. Olai refers to the leaflets of palmyra and suvadi translates to written stock or book. Suvadi may also refer to footprints. Through the writings on these manuscripts, one could deduce the ancient culture, tradition and living style. The earlier practice involved inscriptions on stones, caves, and pottery, but palm leaf manuscripts was more preferred for literary purposes because of its portability.

During the process of writing on palm leaves there is a possibility that there could be typos. Or the poems/pages could be lost as the time goes by. Therefore, it is copied/transcribed to newer palm leaves by disciples in the Gurukulam (monastery). Even though this process is foolproof, there are additional mechanisms to rightly transmit the ancient messages to younger generations is memorizing and reciting the entire volume of the literature. It is interesting to note the anecdotes that not only the students memorize the poems in word by word but also in the inverted order (for example the word 'order' is read inversely as redro). This makes the students and the whole system to pass on the information in a much precise manner without errors. Although Thirumoolar would have been aware of these systems, and have had this kind of disciples, he has used an alternative method to convey the message of his pranayamam as described in Suthiram # 568 (Chapter 5). That is by rephrasing the same message in different words. So just in case there is a copy error in one of the poems or that poem is lost, the other would survive and gets transmitted to the successive generations. Luckily until this point both of his poems (568 and 573) referring to the pranayamam techniques are available/preserved/conserved.

Additionally, this poem gives us a chance to look into the words vaamam, yemam, kaamam, and omam. These words were not used in the poem 568. What is the significance of these words? Vaamam is referred to left nostril. This is a common notation that ida kalai is vaamam. However, the word vaamam also refers to the practice of or the ability to regulate breathing. The person who can effectively regulate breathing is referred as vaami. During conversion/transcription of ancient Tamil into Sanskrit or European words, there is an insertion of S into the beginning of the words. For instance, the word pechu means to speak. This has been a root word for the word speech. Similar to these there are several words where an S is inserted before the first letter (poruthu is to Sport). The word vaami thus became svaami or also spelled as swami, suvami, swamy, or saamy. Adding Su in front of a name is considered adding more laurels to the name. For example, Darshan is vision and adding Su becomes Sudarshan is good vision. Similar to this the one who practices vaamam is vaami, and the person is elevated to even a higher state and becomes SuVaami. Otherwise there is no meaning or other alternative root word for the word Suvami, swamy or sami. Swami refers to God most of the time. However, it is also meant to be for addressing noble people in community, learned ones, foretellers, ascetics and kings. This has become a tradition that several names in India, not just Hindu, but also Christian names have samy. For example, Peria Samy, Muni Samy, Sinna Samy, Mada Samy, Arokiya Samy, Guru Samy, Anthony Samy. Therefore, it is much more meaningful that the word Sami derived from root word Vaami. Vaamam is not just a reference to the ida nostril. But it is the meditative state, also an indication of relaxation, high state of consciousness and best mental prowess. Anyone who could capture this vaama naadi and practices it perfectly becomes vaami/swami. For them it is possible to know the highest wisdom. However, it is the slow path that pranayamam practice takes one into highest level of human being consciousness.

There is a Sithar named Karuvoorar. He is the disciple of Bogar, who in turn is a disciple of Thirumoolar. Therefore, Karuvoorar is the grand-disciple just like grandson of Thirumoolar. From the work of Karuvoorar where he elaborates more on the concept of vaamam, I could deduce that Vaamam is not just the left nostril breathing. It is the the outcome of what the left nostril breathing leads to. There are newer visions in the forehead area as you practice vaamam. Chanting Ang (explained in Chapter 7) is one of the ways that can be used to activate vaama breathing. If you practice vaamam breathing regularly, you can produce more principles that could impact your physical and mental systems. One could understand from Karuvoorar that breathing alone is not sufficient to activate vaamam. This is very interesting. We all think that if we just do a pranayamam physically by changing the breathing pattern everything is going to be achieved. Of course it will have its limited benefits. But if one would elevate the self through pranayamam practice then there is the component that Karuvoorar suggest is the devotion, sincerity, the compassion, a state of love and acceptance of all. It need not be the fear of God. It can be love.

One of the well-known masters of recent times BKS Iyengar says pranayamam without manthiram is incomplete. This is very true. Through manthiram, we condition our mind. We submit ourselves to the greater self, to a greater nature, and to a greater cause. This is the union of self with the ultimate nature. The love and devotion melts the wall between our self and the nature. This state of mind is called Vaamam. We can see the Sakthi herself within us during Vaamam, which means we realize our true ultimate potential. One who achieves this Vaamam is called vaami. Remember vaami is refers to Swami, who is an enlightened person. So when, Thirumoolar says to use Vaamam for inhalation, it is to be understood in this broader perspective. Not just left nostril breathing. It is the main message from this line. This may be another reason why he reworded the Suthiram 568 explained earlier.

Then comes the word yemam. One of the richness of Tamil language is the elaborate meanings that emanate from a single word. The word yemam could be another good example because, it could mean 'special, long, safe, high, esteem, joy, pleasure, wellness and golden. Thiruvalluvar who wrote the literature Thirukkural mentions this word to mean safety (when one is associated with anger then the safety net of relationship surrounding him will reduce to ashes - இனமென்னும் ஏமப்புனையைச் சுடும்). The relationship or the clan or the group around a person is considered as a safety network, that he calls yemam. Therefore yemam in this Suthiram could have multitudinous meanings. I would like to consider the meaning of pleasure, happiness and joy for this word. As you exhale after a breath holding is the time to realize the joy of breath holding. As you breathe out carbon dioxide, you also breathe out the toxic wastes collected from all the tissues of the body. The exhaled air includes not just CO_2 but also several accompanying gases and aerosols that contain compounds/molecules such as sulfur gases, and other metabolic and toxic wastes. Therefore, your diaphragm and lungs get into an euphoric state and took rest as well. Also, the brain waves have been activated become in focused mode. This is the joy that Thirumoolar mentions.

As we carry the burdens of thoughts and past we feel heavy. When we relieve off the burden, when we cast the burden on the Lord, when we share the stories with others our heart feels lighter. Even a good bowel movement in the morning can make the day joyful. One of the Saints in Tamil (called Manickavasakar) sings,

"sitha malam aruvithu sivamakki enai aanda"

(Lord, you removed my impurities in my mind and saved me).

The word malam refers to waste, toxic, remnant, impurity, excrement, and garbage. Sitha malam is the trash held within the mind. He praises the Lord for removing the unwanted from his mind. Once it is removed he becomes Sivam, a nature of Lord himself. So if one gets rid of garbage from any system they are free to enjoy the bliss. Thus, exhalation through the right nostril is the step which opens the windows to the bliss. Also, one would want to consider the generation of brain waves during different steps of this pranayamam. Brain waves are electric currents produced by neurons in different parts of the brain. These brain waves are composed of alpha, beta, theta, and gamma. Each of them have their own range of frequency. Although there is more to be studied about brain waves and their links to pranayamam, there are some earlier studies where the electroencephalogram (EEG) is recorded by placing electrodes on to a person's scalp. Interestingly, researchers have found that pranayamam activates alpha waves refer to a state of relaxation while the subject is in an alert state. Such brain waves are currently stimulated artificially using external electricity as a treatment in some psychosomatic and epileptic patients. It is important to consider that pranayamam practice could promote the brain health through altering the brain waves.

It is possible that each step of TMP (inhalation, holding, and exhalation) would elicit a distinct set of brain waves. Or the exercise as a whole could be the stimulation of such waves. It is to be considered here that several forms of these waves could be produced by external electromagnetic sources, like transcranial magnetic stimulation. However, without the help of external sources one could create such waves by practicing TMP which could reduce symptoms or feelings of anxiety, depression, and mood disorders. This is a great way to maintain mental processes. When one can be joyful with a mere pranayamam practice why would that person require drugs and other addictive behaviors for happiness.

The important phrase in the third line is 'kaamutra pingalai.' Thirumoolar suggests to exhale through right nostril, that is called the pingalai. Why did he use an adjective 'kaamutra' to denote the right nostril. This word describes the pingalai naadi as the one responsible for kaamam, which means desire and lust in general. The right nostril is associated with the sympathetic dominance. For instance, one might notice that sympathetic responses such as anger or aggression lead to the right nostril dominance. Kaamam is a strong emotion that one uses to attach to the goals in life. Achievements and victories are possible through strong desires. Kaamam is fed by the five senses.

Thiruvalluvar, considering the importance of desire and love in life included a section for kaamam in Thirukkural. One of the poems there describes how a young man feels that his all five senses are with the lady he loves, and those five senses enjoy her intimacy (கண்டுகேட்டு உண்டுயிர்த்து உற்றறியும் ஐம்புலனும் ஒண்தொடி கண்ணே உள). I was wondering about the order in which Thiruvalluvar arranged the five senses, which is: sight, hearing, taste, smell, and touch. This order of sensual activation seems to fit this lovely scenario. The mind is fed by all these five senses one by one - in the same order. Why is this order important? Consider how Arunagirinathar, a 15th century saint places the five senses in an order for a yogi who wants to denounce desire and lust. His order is touch, taste, sight, smell and hearing (hey mind, let go the desires following the five senses... ஒழிவாய், மெய் வாய் விழி நாசியொடுஞ் செவியாம், ஐவாய் வழி செல்லும் அவாவினையே). Arunagirinathar's sequence brings a visualization of a yogi first starting detachments with his touch based desires by being alone, then maintains silence and food restriction, then closes his eyes, followed by controlling the desires induced by smell and uses the nostrils for pranayamam, and finally he wins over the hearing too.

The same five senses function in different orders for attachment and detachment. Kaamam is the attachment. This is just opposite to vaamam, denoting the left nostril, that we saw earlier in this chapter. Similar to the person who practices vaamam is called a vaami, the person who practices kaamam is called a kaami. That is why Parvati, the lady who loves Siva is called Sivakaami. For those who want to denounce all desires they need to have an attachment on the one who is detached from everything, says Thirukkural (பற்றுக பற்றற்றான் பற்றினை). That is why Parvati destined her desires towards Siva so she can eventually get detached. Thus, kaamam is a powerful emotion that can be useful to focus on what our desires are. Therefore one needs to cultivate the naadi that regulates kaamam. Pingalai naadi is the one responsible for kaamam. Exhalation through pingala naadi will regulate kaamam, Thirumoolar says. According to this exercise when we can activate the naadi correctly and practice inhalation through vaamam (left) and exhalation through kaamam (right) then it will be a way towards finding the truth.

The next concept Thirumoolar refers in this poem is "omathaal ettettu kumbikka unmaiye." Omam is a spice, also called ajwain seeds. But he does not talk about the spice here. He refers to Om chanting. There are several ways one can perform Kumbakam. For instance we could use Om Namasivaya chanting. However, Thirumoolar suggests here to use Om chanting. One might wonder how to chant, and Om may seem to be a chant of short length (of just two maathirai). But one could extend the number of chanting to a higher value. So if one chants eight Om each for two maathirai then it would account for sixteen maathirai for inhalation. Sixty four maathirai for holding would be thirty two times of Om chanting. Finally, it will be sixteen Om chants for exhalation through right nostril. The chanting and counting may seem like a tedious process to coordinate at the beginning. But if one could set a tune or a pace to the chanting then one can use that rhythm to handle the timing without the need of counting. This can be achieved by practice.

Once when I was going to the LOTUS temple in yogaville, for meditation. I got there a bit late because I took a walk through the woods and got distracted a bit. When I realized I may be running late, I had to rush to the LOTUS. As soon as I reached the mediation hall and sat down I realized that my breathing was fast and I was breathing heavily and a bit loudly too. I was concerned that the people around me could hear my breathing sound and that it might disturb them in their meditation. The twelve noon bell rang for the beginning of the meditation. I cannot keep on breathing heavily and loud anymore. So I controlled the breathing so it can flow slowly. At that instance something struck me; I started saying Om within my mind and tune it to the sound and to the speed of the breath. Every inhalation every exhalation sounded like Om. The ups and downs of the breath during each breathing cycle could be visualized as waves. The motion of my own breath sounded like Om chanting. This helped me to control the heavy breathing within one or two minutes and helped me to enter into meditative stage. This was a great moment of realizing how manthiram such as Om chant could be superimposed to breathing style or frequency, and how breathing could be a route to meditation.

Now let us focus on the last word 'unmaiye' which means 'that is the truth.' Thirumoolar refers pranayamam is the promising path to finding the truth. Every religion every enlightened soul, and every seeker is looking for the truth. Truth is the only thing that is stable, certain and often hidden. That is the light. We search for it the whole life. It is the search for eternal bliss. It is the search for a life without the fears, darkness, worries, and mortality. The Sanskrit slogam that we sing in yogaville from the Bṛhadaraṇyaka Upaniṣad (1.3.28.) says

Asato Maa Sad-Gamaya

Tamaso Maa Jyotir-Gamaya

Mrtyor-Maa Amrtam Gamaya

(Translation: Lead us from unreal to real; lead us from darkness to the light; lead us from fear of death to knowledge of immortality). This is the journey every human being is looking towards either knowingly or unknowingly. We move from place to place desire to desire, and goal to goal. Not satisfied in anything, and not sticking to anything for a long time. Our mind keeps on asking "Is this you wanted forever?" We see a beautiful mobile phone with all the wonderful features of memory, style, apps, ability to connect, store, sync etc. We look for the best place and price to buy, we go to the store, it is not available that day; we go again and again, several trips, several hours of waiting, several hours of searching on the internet, reading about it, gathering and sharing information about the fine details of that phone with all the friends in your WhatsApp contact, and in person. You worry if you would ever get that phone. One fine day you buy your dream phone. You have it right in your hand. You enjoy playing with it, exploring all that your new phone could do for you. You ask a question to find direction to your next door, meaning of life, distance from moon to earth, and the best restaurant to eat your favorite sandwich. Now, after a week you do not have the same excitement like you had in the first day. It fades away. Your mind now drifts to another fantasy. Another material. It is always on the go with new materials, wishes, and desires. None of these materials could make us contented constantly, and eternally.

So, what is the solution? What is the one that is always blissful. It is the truth. There are several pathways to achieve it. Every religion, philosophy, and culture talks about it. Multiple rivers flow into the same ocean. Several roads run into the same destination. Likewise, all the world philosophies talking about attaining this heightened awareness. Thirumoolar says pranayamam is the route to achieve this. Pranayamam could lead to the enlightenment to understand the ultimate truth. Let pranayamam lead your journey to attain truth/enlightenment.

CHAPTER 11

NO DEATH

Original Version (Tamil)

இட்டது அவ்வீடு இளகாது இரேசித்துப்
புட்டிப் படத்தச நாடியும் பூரித்துக்
கொட்டிப் பிராணனும் அபானனும் கும்பித்து
நட்ட மிருக்க நமனில்லை தானே.

Transliteration

    Ittadhu avveedu ilahaadhu resithu

    Putti padathasa naadiyum poorithu

    Kotti pirananum apaananum kumbithu

    Nattam irukka namanillai thaane.

Translation

The home where the soul is kept won't give up (loosen) if you exhale, and then inhale as the ten naadi (idakalai, pingalai, suzhumunai, singuvai, purudan, kandhari, athi, alambudai, sangini, kuhu) are completely engaged. Practice the breath-holding with the inhaled pranan, without exhaling (retaining the apana), and stay up right, then there is no death.

First of all, it is a very bold statement to say that there won't be any death. Death is brought by the demigod Yaman, also called Naman. He is the one who sends out his fellows as soon as one is born, to retrieve the life at the expiry date! It takes our life time for them to reach us as they travel on a slow walking buffalo. Well, if this story is true, theoretically, everyone born on the same day should die on the same day. But the speed of the buffalo is regulated by your own actions or Karma. That is the reason why all the buffalos do not walk in the same speed! Whether it is slow or fast, death is inevitable But for Thirumoolar to say that there is no Yaman and no death, then it must be researched upon to understand what he might have really meant.

It looks to me that Thirumoolar does not refer to physical death here. The word Yaman or Naman could indicate that it is something associated with one's self - me (Yaman) or us (Naman). Death lives with us. Just like the day and night are the part of the day, darkness and brightness are part of the same lamp, like pranan and apanan are two contrasting types of breathing, like growth and recession are appearances of the same moon, so is the life and the death within the same person. When the spirit is down we feel like dead inside. When a tragedy strikes, we feel our heart freezes. We feel a void that there is no Siva (Jivan/seevan/life) dwelling within us anymore. There is no energy to do even the normal day to day tasks. Even if we think we are living, our body's vital functions are still happening, we feel we are without any energy, we are not far from spiritual death. We do have expressions in every language and culture to express that we do not have any life/spirit/ energy to function. In contrast, when we are filled with energy, when we are fully occupied with uplifting spirit, then we think that the life is springing from within us, like a fountain. We are full of energy. This is life. This tells us life and death are happening within us every single moment.

Thirumoolar knows that every birth must end up in death. But he also knows that living does not mean neither mere carrying the body nor just breathing and counting birthdays on the facebook. Life means living as a whole with complete vitality without feeling like a dead spirit. This is one way of interpreting it, i.e., living with full vitality of the spirit, and living a whole life with lot of energy, so that there is no dead space in our lifetime.

The other meaning could be that there is no death to the body itself. However, achieving eternal physical body may not be possible for everyone, including trained Yogis. That is why he has written poems on how to bury a Yogi, what procedures to be followed in the burial including the details of items one needs to put along with the body, how to position the body, the hands and legs too. Thus, he does not speak about the physical body. Rather Thirumoolar seems to speak about the transformation of the physical body into a spiritual body that never dies. He speaks in detail about how our spirit travels after death. i.e., the spirit will go to sun, the moon, reunites with the ancestors and then goes to dwell in the stars. To me it looks so revealing that we normally say such and such person (most often our beloved relatives) is the star blinking up there in the night sky. For example, the Sapta Rishi Mandalam, a group of seven stars (great dipper) is believed to represents seven great saints. Similarly, Arundhathi is another star, known for stability – normally associated with wedding ceremonies.

The stories behind stars are fascinating in all cultures. There are 27 stars referred in Tamil astronomy. These stars are assigned specific names and said to interact with the earth just like the sun and moon. Each day is said to be specific for 1-2 stars as there are 27 stars and more than 27 days in a month. Astrology uses the position of these stars and planets during the birth and determine/predict the life path of a person. Thus, it looks like stars could be considered as collective energy where the spiritual energy after leaving the body is destined to. They use this energy to lit themselves. It may be that every soul should attain certain level of energy to reach the stars. If not they could be recycled to be born again, as new being, until the soul is cultivated to attain higher spiritual energy. This seems to me a part of the grand plan. That is why the yoga philosophy says jivatma (the living beings, like humans) combining with paramatma (the Oneness that expands for ever). Both jivatma and paramatma are part of the same thing. This is the transformation of the perishable physical body to imperishable light body. This is a way of using the spiritual energy in this birth and feeding it into the ever expanding universal energy.

Thirumanthiram and other Sithar anecdotes talk about the body of light. Is it the one that feeds into the stars? The universe is constantly expanding, recycled, gain momentum, and spread. Science says that the galaxies are newly born and expanding. The word Brahman or Pramman or Paraman referring to the god of creation, means the one who is spread. The word 'para' refers to expanded, and widespread. Thus, there is no death to the spiritual 'life' or 'being.' The belief system on reincarnation believes that if the spiritual body does not attain a greater strength and elevation, then it cannot reach the stage of 'light body' and therefore will be born again as a different being. The universe is our home. It is our greater home. Home for everyone. Either it be up in the sky as stars, or as plants in a garden, the souls share the same common universe. Their energy level may be different. Their current position could be different, but in the grand scheme of things, they all move towards the main goal and expanding the universe. Every system has the miniscule universal energy system within itself. Say it be the planetary revolution around the sun and stars similar to electrons around the atomic nucleus. As we are build up with atoms, we have the same principles driving us just like the universe. This is said in Siddha philosophy as "pindathil andam, and andathil pindam" (body within the universe, and universe within the body). So, how does the practice of pranayamam in this perishable physical body help attaining higher spiritual energy that would elevate us to the permanent light-bodied stars? Remember the five kottam again (physical body, breath, mind, wisdom, and bliss). The more time we linger in the outer orbits/layers the more energy we lose and die out. Use the breathing to transcend to the inner core. The mantle is the bliss core. Feed the mantle with all the energy from the outer orbits. That will elevate one to the permanent light body.

One may say, "Well, I do not care about light body and permanence. Is there anything for a normal healthy life in this poem? "Yes. What if this poem is about the physical body and keeping it as long as it is healthy and livable? The first line says that

"Ittadhu avveedu ilahaadhu" means that the home (physical body) where the soul is placed won't lose its temper/strength/stamina/toughness. This is the opening message of this poem. Then he goes on to describe the conditions or the rules or procedures to achieve this. They are: We exhale first, then inhale as all the ten naadi (explained below) bulge/fill completely, perform Kumbakam (breath holding), by keeping or piling up the Pranan and apanan, and stay upright/in the middle (middle also could mean suzhumunai naadi).

We have seen in the previous chapters that inhalation is an important step during pranayamam, also for the normal life, of course. In this poem, he defines inhalation to be done by bulging or filling in all the ten naadi – what are those ten naadi? They are:

Ida naadi that runs from right toe to the left nostril

Pingala naadi that runs from left toe to the right nostril

Suzhumunai – from the tail bone to the crown of the head, running through all the chakras, originating from the mooladharam to sahasrathalam. It is also said that suzhumunai is the balanced state of equal ida and pingala naadi.

Singuvai – that is encompassing all the organs in the nasopharyngeal and laryngeal areas or the visuthi chakaram. Specifically, this controls and coordinates the breathing, swallowing and speech.

Purudan – is the one that controls the right eye

Kandhari – the one controlling the left eye. Both the left and right eye naadi control the blinking, rotation, visual sense, sleep and awake states.

Athi – the one controlling hearing through the right ear.

Alambudai – controls the left ear.

Sangini – this is the one that controls the genitourinary organs' activation. This can be linked to the Swathittana Chakaram.

The 10th naadi is Kuhu – that controls the defecation related activities.

During the practice of naadi sutthi or alternate nostril breathing when you watch closely, after complete exhalation and during the beginning of the inhalation you could sense the two ear naadi are stimulated. I see the stimulation of the naadi through a twitch (lasts less than a second) that could be sensed only when you pay close attention. This is the stimulation or purification or activation that naadi sutthi intends to do. Purification is nothing but allowing new breath, and new energy to follow through that space. Athi and Alambudai are two easily sensed naadi. You might have felt this following another analogy too. When you are not watching and you suddenly hear a sound such as a door click on one side, you will feel the twitching of the ear at that side because of the activation of the motor cortex. Thus, the naadi are not imaginary points, rather they do exist in specific locations and they could be activated through breathing. As we already learned from Thirumanthiram that we can specifically direct our Prana/breath to the place where we send our mind to.

Thirumoolar says 'mann manam engundu, vaayuvum angundu "meaning wherever our mind goes, our breath will be there. Thus, if we think about a place in our body constantly, our pranan enriched and nourished in that part of the body. It is not hard to comprehend; a gymnastic player correctly coordinates his or her mind and sends their neuronal stimulation and energy during the execution of every action/move. That is why, the willpower determines victory in many historic examples. Einstein's corpus callosum was bigger than the normal brain because he was actively engaged in practices that helps him to think, meditate and analyze. A painter's fingers, a pianists arms, a drummers hands, name any, their breath is the one that activates individual local naadi, and sub naadi. The Siddha literature says there are 72,000 naadi in the body.

If it is true that the breath flows through the places where we think, here is a simple exercise! That is to do alternate nostril breathing without using the fingers! Yes, close your eyes. Inhale focusing on the left nostril, your eye balls are rolled naturally towards the left nostril. Pay close attention to the eyeball rotation actions as you inhale slow and steady. At the end of inhalation switch your eyeballs (keep eyes closed) to "see" right side, and focus on the right nostril as you breathe out. You may be surprised that the breath in fact flows through the nostrils where your mind goes and eyes "see." It may not be so obvious at the first instance. But as you practice more and more you will be able to see the coordination.

Naadi do not function without the chakras. Chakras are the major flow channels. Naadi derive messages from the specific chakras near them, just like the regional control centers. For example, Visuthi provides the control actions to Singuvai naadi for a swallowing action. All the 10 naadi are important for our healthy life, for keeping our senses sharp, and to keep our system clean. That is one of the reasons we do naadi sutthi. In early days, the schools/Gurukulam/Palli use breathing exercises before beginning of each class or each ceremony. This means that the energy is flowing through everyone, and within everyone to every part of the body. This gives more support and coherence in the learning process, and removes any misfocus of ideas, energy and workforce. This is critically needed for group activities.

Thus, Thirumoolar talks about the 10 naadi and teaches to fill them with the pranan through a strong and vigorous inhalation step. Remember, to begin doing this type of inhalation, one needs to completely exhale. Philospohically - one cannot fill a non-empty vessel. You need to be empty first before you could begin filling. We should be a dry sponge to absorb water. Lye low to be flown into! Now, back to the technique - the next step after inhalation is to hold the breath, as mentioned in the previous chapters. Here is when the pranan and Apana gases are accumulated within the body, enrich the naadi, and fill all the spaces within our body. Breath holding plays key roles in our health including stimulating some of the brain waves, calming down some of the chaotic ones, increasing the permeability of capillaries, increasing the dilatation of the bronchus, promoting the flow of blood into and out of stagnant miniscule spaces, promotes exchange of gases into those microscopic pores, and siphoning out the toxic wastes accumulated in there.

One of the major benefits of breath holding is that it creates a brief/minor ischemic state which means the tissue in that area, the cells in that space are exposed to a state of reduced oxygen, and increased carbon dioxide. This condition stimulates the cells to activate several survival mechanisms. The cells are now better equipped to withstand the stress. Their ability to face a challenge is boosted. Breath holding is also a key to mobilize stem cells from within the bone marrow and other tissue depots. Researchers have shown that stem cells require a mild hypoxic environment to migrate out of the marrow. Similarly, the differentiation of stem cells into a specialized cell types is also facilitated/aided by the hypoxic environment, just like during the development of a fetus. As you know, the oxygen tension or oxygen availability within the fetus is less than that of the other parts of the mother's body. This reduced oxygen level helps with the specialization of cells much efficiently. Therefore, brief periods of hypoxic conditions during breath holding (Kumbakam) steps is beneficial for replenishing and repairing the constant tissue damage.

If we can take care of the body as mentioned by Thirumoolar in this poem, through this breathing exercise then there is no death to this body. The longer you contain and repair damages, the longer we prevail. The longer will be our healthy life span.

CHAPTER 12

HEALTHY ORGANS AND DIVINITY

Original Version (Tamil)
புறப்பட்டுப் புக்குத் திரிகின்ற வாயுவை
நெறிப்பட உள்ளே நின்மலம் ஆக்கில்
உறுப்புச் சிவக்கும் ரோமம் கறுக்கும்
புறப்பட்டுப் போகான் புரி சடையோனே.

Transliteration
Purappattu pukku thirikindra vaayuvai
Nerippada ulle ninmalam aakkil
Uruppu sivakkum romam karukkum
Purappattu pohaan puri sadaiyone.

Translation
The air that flows in and out and wanders
If one regulates the breath for purification
The body gets a glow and the hair darkens
And the Siva (Lord) that dwells within will not leave you.

Breathing goes in and out constantly. This means the air goes in, travels in, goes out, and travels out. On either side, whether it is within the body or outside the body, the air dissipates, and wanders. We do not know how to regulate it and use the breath as a way to purify our interior. The same pranan could be useful to purify us. If we can achieve it we can have a glowing body with healthy organs, the darken healthy hair, and the Lord (divinity) lives within our body will not depart us.

The message may look similar to the earlier poems. But here is something unique we can derive about the body, the blood flow, the gas exchange and how regeneration works, and how they all could be achieved by regulating the breathing. We know how big the anti-aging industry has been around the globe. The tablets, lotions, creams, herbal extracts and formulations – whatever you possibly could do to the body is all available on the market. Commercials in TV, radio, internet and in malls allure the middle age/elderly population with these products. Similar is the situation for the hair dye/hair transplantation industry. We all love to have head full of healthy hair and feel young just like the middle schoolers. We want to have the body that has the capacity to rejuvenate, to repair, to get rid of all the scars, and to have phenomenally functioning organs in and out. Is this possible or has it ever been possible with any of the drugs or cosmetics that we use, or advertised and available on the market?

The cosmetic industry in India has a strange mindset largely oriented on the skin color. It will use only fair-skinned models, and fair-skinned children for all their product advertisements, whereas their large swath of consumers are brown or dark skinned. They sell 'fairness' creams claiming that you will become a 'fair' (white-like) person if you use their creams. The culture has a severe longstanding discrimination towards dark-skinned population and their feelings. A dark-skinned person does not have a space in the upper society, unless he or she is a celebrity or rich. It is sickening to think about the existence of skin color based social hierarchy. Has it been possible for those drug/cosmetic companies to make Indians to look like Whites? Is it possible for turning the skin color of a person completely with these products? But what is possible is to improve the health of the body, including the skin by making the blood flow well. You notice the face blushes when you are praised in a public space, or on a stage. But the face darkens in shame and stress. Face glows when you laugh, when in intimacy, or having a good time with your friends. What it tells you is that a joyful laughter can stimulate circulation of blood throughout the body, especially through the head/brain. This helps us take care of our thought process in a more positive, happier and lighter manner.

Thirumoolar says in the first two lines that if one could regulate the breath (that normally goes awry) in right place, then the body/organs become red and the hair blackens. There is another way of looking at the 'reddening' of organs or 'blackening' of hair. This means that there is more blood flow to the organs. This could be achieved by another physiological process called hypercapnia. i.e., by mildly increasing the amount of carbon dioxide within the body. When we regulate the breathing frequency, pace or speed, for instance by reducing the number of breaths per minute, or breath-holding, then that induces a mild increase in the building up of carbon dioxide within the body. This increase leads to dilatation of capillaries and bronchus. Imagine what we do when we hold our breath to lift something heavy, or for some other biological processes, we hold the breath and set the mind there, send neuronal stimulation to that spot. This leads to an increased muscle contraction/dilatation that eases up the process in the target organs. This transient hypercapnia is also responsible for the reddening of the face. Of course, excessive hypercapnia along with hypoxia will not be good for health as it might deprive cells of necessary oxygen to function optimally. But a mild hypercapnia would facilitate the flow of blood to the minor capillaries, in addition to large vessels. As the practice continues this will also enhance blood flow through scalp. Poor circulation to the scalp is responsible for greying and baldness. This circulatory insufficiency could affect skin too. The coldest parts in our body are the finger tips, toes, feet and the skins (depending upon where they are). When blood flow is increased through these areas then there will be more energy and nutrients released into these areas, and the toxins are removed efficiently. Therefore, intermittent increase in carbon dioxide is a good way to promote blood flow. When there is a good flow of blood then that part of the body is healthy whether it is skin or scalp or other organs in the body.

Certain foods can promote circulation, for example red pepper. But pepper come with a burning sensation of tongue and possible impact on stomach too. Plus, you can consume only so much in any given time. That is why Thirumoolar is talking about breath holding. When we practice the TMP, we see the breath holding (Kumbakam) is the longest duration. This helps to accumulate more carbon dioxide within the body for the set duration which is the longest of all the three processes – inhalation, holding and exhalation. Even he calculated the exhalation to be twice longer than the inhalation. This helps extending the time of carbon dioxide accumulation.

There is another reason to the breath holding by TMP that could lead to improved health. That is the lymphatic health. The lymphatic system consists of lymph nodes, spleen and the thymus. The blood cells, particularly the ones that are responsible for our immune system and well-being, the white blood cells (WBC) are derived from the precursor cells in bone marrow and move to spleen or thymus where they differentiate further to become specialized B or T cells. These cells circulate via the lymphatic system using the current of lymphatic fluid. The lymphatic fluid contains all the blood components except the red blood cells (RBC). At the tissue level blood capillaries exchange fluids and blood cells with lymphatic system. The lymphatic fluid drains into the venous blood in upper chest (inferior/superior vena cava). The lymphatic flow in humans is not maintained by a pump like the heart. However, in some other animals there is a 'lymph heart' that pumps lymphatic fluid. Humans use the movement of the diaphragm to create pressure changes that aid in lymphatic flow. Breath holding increases thoracic cavity's pressure during Kumbakam. This puts a short pause to the lymphatic flow; a stagnation point. As a result, it increases the pressure within the lymphatic vessels that run via the thorax. When the pressure is released during Resakam (exhalation) this flow is resumed with a faster movement. This can be correlated with stepping onto a water hose. When the foot is on the hose, it blocks the flow and thus causes an increase in pressure within the upstream hose. When the foot is released, water flows again with an increased speed due to the pressure gradient created. Breath holding helps in the regular maintenance of the lymphatic system, flow of cells across all over the body to take care of the immune functions.

The lymphatic system is not only critical to fight germs, but also helpful in removing toxins from the body. These toxins could be the usually accumulated byproducts of metabolism such as uncleared large protein aggregates arising from cellular metabolism. Remember, accumulation of protein aggregates are the major responsible factors for neurodegenerative diseases such as Alzheimer's disease. In addition to natural waste products, we accumulate externally 'added' waste products that get deposited in tissues. These include 4000 plus chemicals that we use or exposed to in our everyday life that are potential carcinogens. Recent data from the year 2016 from the Environment Working Group in the USA clearly indicates that over 420 chemicals are in dangerously high levels in human body as estimated from participants' urine, blood and milk.

Another potential hazardous substance is the Advanced Glycation End products (AGEs) that are present in large quantities in processed food. These AGEs are not easily cleared from the body unless we specifically recruit white cells through the efficient flow of lymphatic fluid. In fact, lymphatic flow could be promoted by some of the asanas such as Sarvanga asana (shoulder stand) or forward bend, head to knee on a chair. As the lymphatic flow from the lower parts of the body could be facilitated by reducing the gravitational force, i.e. lifting the legs. When we need to sit up for a longer time we must engage in breathing exercises. In several ways, it seems like pranayamam helps a Yogi to keep up good physical health when engaged in long periods of sitting in for meditation. Therefore, those whose career/job requires extended sitting should practice some pranayamam exercises.

The last line of the poem says that Lord Siva who has hair that's long as strings won't leave the body. The hair strings may even refer to the naadi within the body. When the breath is regulated then the body will regain its youthfulness as seen by the health of the hair and the skin, and thus the soul will not leave the body.

One might think that the effects caused by yoga breathing are very systemic, and how that could heal a specific disease such as cancer in the breast or in the prostate for example. This is where the current therapies are insufficient. Right now, we talk about targeted therapy or personalized medicine to first analyze the type of mutations that the cancer tissue has, and then treat with the drug or combination of drugs specific for that gene defect. But cancer research since the early 1970s is proving that the targeted therapy may not work. Although it may seem like working, after sometime the cancer comes back with more vigor. Studies on genetic profiling, for instance mutations where the DNA is mutated at various genes to change their function, and gene amplification where the number of times that gene is multiplied within the same genome to enable the extraordinary overexpression of the corresponding protein, are key to understanding the genetic background of the disease. Or there is this another type of aberrant modification called genome duplication where the whole genome condensed within chromosomes is duplicated. i.e., instead of one pair of chromosome the cancer cells end up getting two pairs. This results in loss of normal regulation, means loss of usual control mechanisms on cell growth, survival or cell death. The result is nonstop growth of clones and clones of cells with extreme variations in their ability to grow under different environment. Some cancer cells start differentiating to numerous types of cancer cells. This leads to a situation where one cannot control or treat the cell growth with just one drug. One pathway if blocked, the smart cancer cells use another pathway, and another. The ability of cancer cells to keep growing and surviving destroying the normal tissue space is enormous. With no boundaries to physical location, they migrate to distant tissues, spreading the seeds as a weed, use all the resources within the body, evading the immune response, using up the nutrient sources, and interfering with normal tissue architecture and function.

Can this extreme malady be treated with just one drug? Can this systemic deterioration be cured with one fix? When a car gets into an accident got a broken bumper, airbag deployment, engine damage and physical injury to the driver, all because there was a problem in the brake, will then all be reverted by just fixing the brake? This is the analogy George Cooper, my former division director, and a renowned cardiologist say of heart diseases. This can very well be used for any disease. There is no single fix because the diseases get systemic. When the disease is systemic how should the treatment be? Systemic. Simple, isn't it? There was a joint study from Buck institute and UCLA on Alzheimer's disease. They used a combination of diet, exercise, yoga, sleep hour regulation, and eating time, all properly adhered and monitored. When this happened for a few months they were able to show signals that it could reverse memory loss, a key problem in AD. Similarly, when Dean Ornish combined yoga (aka stress management!), nutrition, exercise and psychological counseling then the heart disease is reversed. Therefore, it is not true that medicines/pills alone can cure diseases, especially chronic illnesses.

Thirukkural says that treatment is successful only when four parts (the patient, doctor, medicine, and the caregiver) work together properly (உற்றவன் தீர்ப்பான் மருந்து உழைச்செல்வான் அப்பால் நாற் கூற்றே மருந்து). What is the responsibility of the patient? The patient needs to create a physical and mental environment and determination to remove the disease from within. We see patients with ultimate positive attitude, controlled behavior in terms of food, exercise, mood, and adherence to medication get better sooner than those in the opposite camp. In fact, patient comes first. The patient is not a passive subject in the treatment process. It is the 25% share for the patient. The next 25% each is the doctor, and then the medicine. The final 25% is the caregiver, who goes through the disease along with the patient. This is holistic wellness explained well over 2000 years ago, by Thiruvalluvar. The word referring to the caregiver here (உழை; uzhai) refers to the heart chakra in music. The musical note 'ma' which is also called madhyamam (uzhai) originates from the heart chakra. It is the center note of the seven notes in Tamil classical music. This tells us that the caregiver should function from the heart center. The caregiver is kind to the patient, understands the disease, and makes connections between all the other three components.

We also can correlate the disease to the type of variant, bold, aggressive, powerful species – often referred to as Asurar (or Asura) in ancient Indian literature. I acknowledge that there is a cultural derogatory use of this term. But in this context I am using it to depict the opposite force in the body. The body has a rhythm, life has a rhythm – this is called suram. Thiruvalluvar says isaipada vaazhthal (இசைபட வாழ்தல்) means living with harmony. Our cells live in harmony. They have a rhythm. Those that do not have rhythm are the A-surars or arrhythmic. They are the evil forces. Those cells that do not have the rhythm are Asurar-like, they grow out of control. Cancer is like Asurar. Hard to defeat. If you kill one, the other will appear, in a different form from a different source. Asurar acquired special power from the same source, Lord Siva, the one who dwells within us. He is the basis of life. He is the one who destroys the old ones and the bad ones, and constructs new ones. His cosmic dance is a symbol of constant transformation that goes on in the universe inside and outside of us. Then how does the mythical story end? Asurar defeated by the goodness. This goodness is a combination of good intention, tactics and time.

Trying to fight with the Asurar-like cancer with equally Asuratic drugs are not going to neutralize the cancer. We need a goodness tool, which is a systemic approach. Of course, the pill has 25% of its share in curing, but the other parts must come together do their job too. This is where yoga comes in again. It is systemic; the effects, markers and targets of yoga are systemic, affecting mind, body and beyond. When one starts with yoga, then the habits on food, drinks, smoking, mood, worries, friendliness, social interactions, and the ability to cope up with stress all come together.

Pranan regulation is the driving force of yogic way of life. When the pranan is regulated within the body, there is no place for illness, disease, and evil forces. The Lord will stay within us – for ever – so long as we love, like, and work on it.

CHAPTER 13

THE LENGTH OF THE BREATH

Original Version (Tamil)

கூடம் எடுத்துக் குடிபுக்க மங்கையர்
ஓடுவர் மீளுவர் பன்னிரெண்டு அங்குலம்
நீடுவர் எண்விரல் கண்டிப்பர் நால்விரல்
கூடிக்கொளின் கோல அஞ்செழுத்தாமே
(கூடிக்கொள்மின் கோல அஞ்செழுத்தாலே)

Transliteration

Koodam eduthu kudipukka mangaiyar

Oduvar neeluvar pannirendu angulam

Needuvar enviral kandippar naalviral

Koodikkolin kola anjezhuthaame

(Koodikolmin kola anjezhuthaale).

Translation

There are two ladies living in this house

They run in and out at a length of twelve angulam

Extension for eight counts and holding for four counts

If one would like, embrace this practice with the help of the fiver letters.

I want to repeat one thing: there are more than one interpretations! Thirumanthiram is like an art that contains a scenic formation in. Everyone sees the cloud. However, one finds a sheep, the other one sees it as a sign of rain, and the other one looks at it a hindrance to the bright sun rays on a breezy morning. What I see in this poem first is a Suthiram for a pranayamam method. I will also explain the other possible meanings below in this chapter.

The normal length of the breath is twelve angulam (approximately 36 centimeters, because one angulam is approximately three centimeters). If we imagine attaching a colored object to mark the tip of the breath that goes out as we exhale, and measure how long it travels until the end of the exhalation process, it would have traveled to the distance of twelve angalam. This is the ideal length of breathing. But it may not be the length that we normally breathe. This is shortened because we do not pay attention, or bring our awareness to the breathing process. When we breathe consciously we tend to extend the breathing for a longer period of time, by engaging our abdomen and chest, then we will be able to attain the full length of twelve angulam.

Breathing deep and slow has been emphasized in Thirumanthiram in several places. To facilitate attaining this length there is an exercise called Savithri Pranyamam. Although the name of this pranayamam or its measurements is not given in this poem, I see a good correlation between the two here. This pranayamam is done in the following way with the help of the Phrase: Na-Ma-Si-Va-Ya (five letters in Tamil). Say this word eight times within your mind and count with your fingers. At the end of full inhalation hold the breath for four counts of Na-Ma-Si-Va-Ya. Then exhale for eight counts of chanting. After complete exhalation, hold the breath for four counts of Na-Ma-Si-Va-Ya. At this step you basically wait before you take the next inhalation. The sequence of the whole exercise goes like this: 1) inhale, 2) hold, 3) exhale, and 4) hold, and repeat the cycle starting from step 1.

This exercise helps to extend the breathing and increases the ability to hold your breath. We always rush into the breathing process. It is because of all the emotions that we go through, and the thought processes that fly by do have an effect on our breathing. When you hear a very soothing sound of spa music or a chanting, your breathing slows down. On the other hand, a hip-hop song could make your heart rate increase. Interestingly, music has a great influence on our breathing as well. When we sing or hear a soothing, melodious, slow pace music then the breathing extends and vice versa. Research studies show that music calms mind, reduces heart rate, reduces blood pressure and slows down the breathing rate. It is amazing how some songs fit or overlap with the flow of our breath. Heart beat becomes the tempo during the music. When the breathing rate is slower, the heart rate also dips. That's why philosophers like Thiruvalluvar say there is no great gift that philanthropy and a harmonious life.

When we have harmony with our breathing and mind, we are one with ourselves. When that happens it could bring several others into the same fold. Everyone walks into becomes one with us. We do see music is a great tool to unite people at multiple levels. A composer who can find the harmony of the soul becomes successful in capturing the attention of the audience (when I write this I think of my favorite composer, Ilayaraja). When we listen to such music, our heart beats in sync with the music, and the breathing too gets aligned with the music. The breathing technique given in this poem helps one to achieve the slow and steady breathing which could have a significant impact on calming down our anxious mind just like listening to soulful relaxing music.

The other meaning to this poem is related to how the breathing gets shortened as we age, especially when one not paying attention to the breathingShortened breathing makes us breathe more number of times in a minute. The breathing is shallow, the diaphragm, the intercostal muscles, and the lungs do not work to their fullest elastic potential. The result is insufficient circulation of air throughout the body and hence accumulated stress in both mind and body. As the first line of the poem says, there are two women that live in this hall (body). Thirumoolar refers to the breathing through two – the ida and pingala naadi. Those two women can run and retract (or run back and forth) for twelve angulam. The length of this twelve angulam breath will reduce when we do not pay attention to this process; the length of the breath gets reduced to eight angulam by involuntary restriction of four angulam. This reduction of four angulam breathing could be improved when we can perform the breathing with mindfulness. We can voluntarily extend or deepen the breathing by the help of chanting the five letter manthiram (mantra) Na Ma Si Va Ya. This is an effective methodology for extending the breathing to the original twelve angulam. The other meaning for the last line is that if we do extend the breathing to twelve angulam, then we could live long as the five letter word Na Ma Si Va Ya itself. This chant is multi-dimensional. Some see this as a chant that eliminates any future rebirths. Some chant this to relieve from mental and physical afflictions. And, some sing this chant to express their love and devotion to the Lord. Whatever may be the case, this chant has a beauty, and Thirumoolar says that the life becomes as beautiful as the chant itself.

Na Ma Si Va Ya is one of my favorite chants. I chant this while driving. One can vary this chant by adding an Om in front of it. If one likes to make it as a praise of Jesus it is quite possible: Ye Su Ve Na Ma. Here Yesuve means Oh, Jesus. Nama is praising. These are similar sounds, and may have similar benefits. It does not matter which religion, which God or what chant. All we need is chanting of some sort. Prayers at the LOTUS founded by Swami Satchidananda has chants incorporating several religions from around the globe. I love chanting all of them. I want to mention something about how vocalization impacts our biology. I noticed something interesting with salivary stimulation in chanting Om, Namasivaya and Om-Namasivaya. In my practice, I observed Om chanting alone, without adding any other syllables predominantly produces watery saliva. This could mean that the major salivary glands activated are the parotid glands. This is the one which produces watery saliva. Continuous repetition of Namasivaya produces kind of a more mucous type saliva. This could be activating the sublingual and submaxillary glands. When we combine Om and Namasivaya all the three types of salivary glands are stimulated and the saliva seems to be a mixture of watery and mucous. It will be very interesting to measure and compare the biochemical components in each type of saliva.

Thirumoolar has reiterated the importance of chanting the five letters (Namasivaya) or the single letter (Om) in several places throughout Thirumanthiram. It appears from this poem that the five-letter chanting with controlled breathing has some key effects on extending or maintaining the functions of the lungs, and of course has the added benefits on the health of the mind.

CHAPTER 14

NO DAY NO NIGHT

Original Version (Tamil)
பன்னிரெண்டு ஆனைக்குப் பகலிரவு உள்ளது
பன்னிரெண்டு ஆனையைப் பாகன் அறிந்திலன்
பன்னிரெண்டு ஆனையைப் பாகன் அறிந்தபின்
பன்னிரெண்டு ஆனைக்குப் பகலிரவு இல்லையே

Transliteration
Pannirendu aanaikku pahaliravu ulladhu
Pannirendu aanaiyai paahan arindhilan
Pannirendu aanaiyai paahan arindhapin
Pannirendu aanaikku pahaliravu illaiye.

Translation
There are twelve elephants – they have day and night
The mahout doesn't know these twelve elephants
When he comes to know about the twelve elephants
Then the twelve elephants do not have day and night.

To experience the beauty of this poem let me briefly touch upon how environmental factors have a strong influence on biological systems. Realization of the "time" is the most powerful factor driving the development and/or aging process. There are certain biological processes such as the circadian rhythm (circadian clock) within the body that senses the time and sends signals accordingly. The genes that control the circadian rhythm are expressed differentially in the day and night. The cells within a specific region of the brain might be able to sense whether it is a night or a day. This region of the brain is called the suprachiasmatic nuclei (SCN). SCN receives inputs from the sensory organs about the light and regulate the metabolic functions through neurohormones. There is another cycle within the body called the feeding cycle. This is similar to the circadian rhythm but depends upon feeding-refeeding cycles. Interestingly the feeding cycle also has an influence on the SCN region of the brain. Some of the proteins involved in the feeding cycle get activated as soon as we eat, and then come to basal levels (resting state) during fasting period. It is known from several studies that calorie restriction leads to longevity.

In an interesting experiment, when the fruit fly were fed lesser than a normal diet, they were found to live at least 10% longer compared to the ones that were fed unconditionally. Studies have also shown that inhibitors of the proteins involved in feeding cycle (our eating habits) can also enhance longevity. For example, rapamycin (a drug produced by bacteria as an antibiotic) when administered to lab mice was found to inhibit one of the crucial pathways involved in the feeding cycle. These mice lived longer compared to the untreated control group. A famous quote by Saint Vallalar would be apt here: "Stay alone, stay hungry, and stay awake (தனித்திரு, பசித்திரு, விழித்திரு)." This is a pithy maxim not just for saints, but also for common men who need to trigger his self-awakening. Too many wonderful ideas flow naturally into our minds when we are able to control our hunger. As a result, we become attuned to the frequency of the universe and become a reservoir for all the five fundamental elements – air, land, water, fire and space - that govern the cosmic space. Let the noble thoughts come to us from every direction – as nicely quoted by Swami Vivekananda. Therefore, either through calorie restriction or behavioral practices such as pranayamam, one could exert an effect on the SCN to alter the circadian rhythm. The same SCN has a profound influence on aging as well. Impaired SCN function leads to faster aging. While the role of SCN is still beginning to be understood, studies suggest that SCN could be regulated by our activities/behavior to control the outcomes. Because pranayamam has a strong influence on the mind and the body, I envision that it also has the potential to regulate SCN and thus the circadian rhythm.

The twelve elephants mentioned in this poem can be interpreted in a couple of different ways. For example, it could be the twelve packets of breath. Breathing is inhaled and released in bundles or packets (similar to how light and sound waves travel). The coordinated muscular movement associated with breathing is nonlinear in nature: they go up and down in small waves with a small pause in the middle. If you inhale counting twelve you can feel how each count is filling up in fractions. In the same way you can count twelve fractions as you exhale.

There is a breathing exercise called the "Four Parts Breathing," where the the inhalation component is divided into four parts or fractions with no exhalation in between. It is like taking four small steps to climb one staircase. In the same way, exhalation is carried out in four steps (without any inhalation in between). This helps in inhaling and exhaling to the fullest capacity. Now imagine that each breath is segmented into twelve parts and each part is contributing to the overall vitality. All these twelve fractions make up one full inhalation and one full exhalation. This helps to build up or gain control of fullest breathing capacity. By engaging our abdomen and chest in this exercise, one can reduce the number of breaths per minute.

The count twelve also makes me wonder about the twelve hours that makes a day and night. Those twelve hours are each one elephant. One could bring in all the other significant twelve collections like the twelve months in Tamil calendar, and later in English (remember, the Western calendar had only ten months in the beginning; July and August were added much later into the calendar), the twelve rasis or the group of stars that align with the movement of the moon (can be the like the zodiac sign).

However, the key message that Thirumoolar conveys here is related to how the time can be forgotten or eliminated when one engages in yoga breathing. During multiple pranayamam training sessions, I have seen people wondering how quickly the class was over! Time flies so fast when we are engaged in breathing exercises or any mindfulness practices for that matter. What does it tell you? Time is perceived by mind too. Whatever is denoted by those twelve elephants – it is the one that controls our time sense. Being aware of those elephants is a strategy to get out of the day-night cycles.

When human mind becomes impervious to no day-night cycles, then aging process can be controlled. In a different poem, this is what Thirumoolar conveys about the day-night life cycles: "I was in" this body for millions where both night and day cannot be perceived (இருந்தேன் இக்காயத்தே எண்ணிலி கோடி; இருந்தேன் இராப்பகல் அற்ற இடத்தே). This he says when he refers to being with his Guru. This may not just mean that he was in the body for that long years. It may be that there is something within the body which is so enriched and was unable to make the distinction between day and night. Can the millions indicated in the poem could mean millions of cells? Or the type of cells that distinguishes day and night? Or did he regulate all those cells which eventually become insensitive to day and night? I like the last one: that is, through the awareness of those powerful twelve elephants, the group of cells within the body attained a unique state and are liberated from the elements that control circadian rhythm, aging process, and feeding/refeeding cycles. They are not controlled by routine day-night cycles. Don't you think a unique state that helps you produce neurohormones whenever you want through regulation of breathing is interesting?

We know people living in cold climate regions (for example, Tromsø city in Norway) are deprived of sunlight for several months - a.k.a, polar nights. As a result, they go through a state of depression and/or mood disorders. To circumvent this, some take nutritional supplements such as melatonin that could help manage their transient symptoms. If one could produce these compounds through breathing exercises, then it would have strong positive effect on cells whether the ambience is day or night. Slow-cycling cells, i.e., cells that divide and produce daughter cells in a slow fashion has a long survival time. Human cells depending upon the organ type have varying life spans. On the other hand, a bacterial cell replicates within 20-30 minutes, and completes its life within a day. It would be intriguing to identify the factors that determine the life expectancy of different cell populations within the human body. Say, organs like heart and brain do not replace their cells as often as the skin, or liver or immune cells do. It could be dependent upon circadian gene expression, and nutrition availability, or potentially upon breathing regulation. The more nutrition we provide we crank up some type of cells' growth and division. We build more muscles and fat which in turn it makes more machinery to tackle the workload. Increased growth also means increased metabolic rate. I see people eating so much and exercising so much. Both could be good in their view. They love over-feeding themselves. Also they feel good when they run six miles the next morning. And they are ready for subsequent feeding cycle. A system that produces its own factors to handle feeding/fasting cycle without much external influence is an efficient system. This could be something like energy efficient and good to the environment. It doesn't consume a lot and doesn't excrete a lot. There is much less waste products. At the same time, the system is optimized to do good to the self and to the world.

Those twelve elephants also could be the breaths that extend for twelve angulam as we saw in the previous chapter. The twelve elephants are powerful. Elephant symbolizes hidden power. Depending on the situation, it stays calm or aggressive.. However, it can be brought under control by a mahout. Famous mythological characters including Hanuman and Veeman display elephant-like strength.

Does the million elephants mentioned in the poem actually refer the elephants? Or, is it a euphemism? One explanation could be that he indirectly means the cells that did not see light of the day. They are as powerful as elephant, nourished by the breathing. Those cells can be controlled and conditioned to lose the sense of day and light using breathing. A regulation in breathing produces factors that can activate or stimulate a variety of emotions including elation, and enlightenment to the cells. These cells lose their ability to sense time. Just like the cows in the Kovardhana mountains giving copious amount of milk after listening to the wonderful flute of Kopalan, their cowherd. Ko means cow. Cows can be considered as the five senses within us. These five cows do not have a proper cowherd. When there is a Kopalan, a good cowherd, there is a lot of milk. Control the five senses. Easy? Not much. But with controlled mind, with Kopalan, it is easy. Kopalan cannot control the cows without a flute – the breath. Flute is the breath. Kopalan is the mind. Where is the melody? Breath cannot be melody. Regulation of the breath is the melody. Pranayamam is the way to produce melody from the flute. The five cows are the five senses. Milk is what we gain – it could be the nourishment to the mind and to the body – a way to enlightenment. Kopalan is depicted dark in Hindu mythology. The mind could be dark. It can take care of the cows, the senses. Kopalan loves milk, curd, and butter. Kopalan herds the cows. The cows feed Kopalan. This is a system of symbiosis. Beautiful melody flows in that hilly meadow. Water, and milk flow in the meadow, and all the angels walk through. Kopalan takes care of the cows. There is this tiger and deer next to each other drinking from the same pond. There is no day or night. Mahout knows how to control those twelve elephants. The elephants made the whole entirety a beauty. The blissful serene eternity.

Om Namasivaya
Om Shanthi
ஓம் நமசிவாய
ஓம் சாந்தி

FURTHER READING

1. Tirumanthiram. In: Tirumanthiram English Translation of Tamil Spiritual Classic by Saint Thirumular. Hawaii: Himalayan Academy Publications. https://www.himalayanacademy.com/view/tirumantiram

2. www.PranaScience.com

2. திருமந்திரம். விளக்கவுரை: ஞா. மாணிக்கவாசகன், உமா பதிப்பகம், சென்னை

Made in the USA
Middletown, DE
14 November 2023

42719728R00071